RENEWED YOU

HOW TO LOSE WEIGHT AND ANTI-AGING ALTOGETHER BY FOOD AND WORKOUTS (FOR PEOPLE FROM 7 TO 77 YEARS OLD)

For all who have body shame like I was

By Thailan Chi

Preface

It's time for you. Most people are excited about anti-aging without surgery because they want to look younger than friends at the same age for as long as they can. It's the desire from most people (especially women) from all the time (ancient, now and future). So, how do we let time not age our faces for as long as possible? Are there any simple methods we are able to choose to continue all lives with beautiful faces with joy and consistency? Can we always look like we are 20 even when we're going to reach 30 or maybe 50 years old? I'd like to share with you all my experiences about losing weight happily and how I keep my face look like 20 years old without surgery. I hope these little tips based on my experience for years will be helpful to all of you

1

who are suffering body shame like I was. You will be free from negative thoughts, such as, will my skin be ugly after going on the diet without working out? Or, why I look like an old lady at the age of 20? All of your answers will be found here. Stay tuned with this book and give it a shot.

Table of Contents

Chapter 1. Natural face lift

1. The gift of nature

Besides making you fat, sugar is the main factor makes your skin go worse.

A study[1] published in the journal of the American college of nutrition, *in which researchers studied the diets of 435 adults living in different countries, found that those who consumed more fish, olive oil and legumes were less prone to wrinkles than those who ate more meat, butter, high fat dairy and sugar.*

Vegetables and fruits are sweet to those who have eliminated sugar and other sweeteners from their diets. It simply takes time for the body to readjust after you have eliminated them. Substitute a protein-based snack whenever you do have a craving for sweet. Your body will thank you and you will be more energetic. As for me, I keep a habit of eating cucumbers and tomatoes everyday to keep my skin bright.

----

[1] Allison Tannis, M.S., R.H.N. FEED YOUR SKIN, STARVE YOUR WRINKLES:Eat Your Way to Firmmer, More Beautiful Skin with 100 Foods That Turn Back the Clock. 2009.

One of the most effective egg-based foods I've tried that helps increase collagen and improve skin texture is free ranged eggs steeped in wild honey. A food rich in magnesium, vitamin e, protein, minerals, etc. which helps you improve your skin naturally.

How to make eggs steeped in honey:

Ingredient:

- 1 glass jar
- Free ranged eggs (quantities according to jars)
- Wild honey

Instruction:

- Take only egg yolks. Put them into glass jars. Steep in honey. Put the lid on tight.
- Put the jars in the fridge. You can start eating 1 egg a day after 1-2 days of steeping. Honey can make egg glutinous quickly. I eat like 'inteval eating' (eat 1 egg every 2 day). The honey only brings good quality within 1 month so be careful to change them.
- You should eat in the morning (because it is rich in many nutrients)

Tip: this is food for your skin, improving your collagen. But, you must change the honey after one month. So, you should keep enough eggs and honey in your jars enough for one month.

For the drink to boost my new day, I enjoy "warm water boom" with honey and turmeric. Drinking it every morning right after waking up and you'll see how does it boost you all day long. Instruction:

- Half a glass of warm filtered water
- Add 1 slice or just some drops of lemon juice if you'd like.
- 1-2 tsp of turmeric powder. You should choose a brand called turmeric powder.
- Also add 1-2 tsp of wild honey (depending on your glass size)

Drinking warm water in the morning will *kick start the liver and gallbladder and digestive function. This is alkalising and helps with fat metabolism also*[2]. I have been drinking this way every morning since I was 26 years old to prevent aging. If you drink turmeric everyday like I said, you will see how it benefits your skin. It takes

---

[2] Rick Hay. The Anti Aging Food & Fitness Plan. 2016.

several months to see significant improvement but it is worth waiting. So do it consistently and you'll never regret it.

For a little more scienfic details, the mixture of turmeric and honey would make it become one of the most powerful antibiotics every physicians should recommend you to drink. Turmeric is the ancient ingredient which appeared in almost powerful anti-aging products such as face cream, drink, medical treatment, etc., it produces curcuminoids. This is a very strong anti-oxidant which is good for the skin and it has *antiseptic, antibacterial, anti-fungal and anti-inflammatory properties* which fight against wounds and allergies in one musical note! And honey is also proved to exert *antioxidant, antimicrobial, anti-inflammatory, antiproliferative, anticancer, and antimetastatic effects*. That's why the drink has two of efficient ingredients has the effects we want exactly on our skin.

2. Double cleansing

I want to tell you a story about my skin years ago when I was a teen. It was years of naivety and cruelty altogether. I was naive at the time and those years were cruel.The only one thing I knew was trying my best to study in school for not being the "left behind friend" in my classes. My friends always told me that they thought my skin was "the punishment of God" because it was full of acne covering my whole face. It was like the hide of an unknown animal, nearly pulled out from the barrel of oil. It was my deepest insecurity all those years. In recent years, my skin became better thanks to some tips of food mentioned in this book. Aside from turmeric drink and breathing techniques, one of the most compulsory things you must do each day is wash your face. You can wash 2-3 times per day although I suggest 2. However, face cleansing is not a simple step to do. It contains two important steps you must remember if you want clean, smooth, and glowing skin. I used to take one step for washing my face and it was the biggest mistake I ever made. My skin produced more oil than ever before. I didn't know how to use face cleansing oil to wash my face. After a couple of years of experimenting, I'd like to tell you that every woman needs to double cleanse their face regardless their type of skin 2 times per day, once in the morning and once in the evening before going to bed.

Step 1: use branded baby oil for massaging for 1-2 minutes all over the corners of your face. Pour it on clean hands and lightly put it on your face. Slowly and tenderly massage onto your face like you are touching an egg. Do not put too much pressure on your face because it can hurt and damage your sensative skin, or you can apply it on your face equally and leave it for 1-2 minutes.

Step 2: mix your oil on your face with a little water to make them become a compound. With water on your hands, mildly massage on your face. Leave it for 1 minute.

Step 3: you can wash your face with your daily cleanse foam. I use foam cleansing for my sensitive oily acne prone skin in recent years, and I got hooked on it. It's like toppings put on drinks that deeply wash my skin but do not weigh down on my skin. You should wash your skin after 2-3 minutes. That time is suitable for the foam works on your skin. When your face is clean, pamper it gently with soft towel until it's dry.

I can guarantee after 3 super simple steps of double cleansing, you'll feel refresh inside out on your face.

Tip: don't touch your skin all day. Just let it free of touching.

3. Use retinol or tretinoin

My acnes almost cleared from my face thanks to retinol panacea. Besides working out myself, retinol and double cleansing are main factors make me feel relieved in some recent years after a long time suffering acnes and ugly skin through adolescent to mature. Retinol 0.025% is the first step you should try for a better skin. It can cure almost every skin problems like acnes, wrinkle, sagging skin, etc. I used to use retinol 2-3 nights before going to bed and then increased the frequency of using it slowly when my skin was still unfamiliar with it. If your skin is sensitive like mine, you should use it once a week and then increase slowly with care. Always use a quantity of a pea because it works depending on how you use, not on the amount.

When your face gets accustomed to retinol every day or you think it's time to try tretinoid for the better treatment, try it. It is a stronger cure than retinol. Or you can continue using retinol if you feel bad about tretinoid. It's up to your skin. They both can fight anti-aging, acne and more. But you must be careful when using one of them for the most effective results you hope to achieve. Always a "pea-size" amount and apply it at night on your face. Using more will not help in the anti-aging way, but it can lead to damaging your face. It's sensitive to sunlight, so you must care for your skin in the day by using sunscreen or making an protection for it by wearing a hat, thick face mask, veil or shawl. You can use both retinol or tretinoin only at night without strong electric light. They are likely to mitigate effects if they face strong lights too.

If you are consistent and careful, I'm sure you'll receive the dream skin one day.

4. Live in harmony with people around you

We tend to be friends with nature for a better life and relief. But we also tend to forget how to live happier in today's society due to busy lifestyle. I realized that one of the most efficient ways to live happier is that we live in harmony with people around us. Not try to be their enemy or foe, rather try to be friendlier and sympathize. Anger and all sorts of negative feelings do not only affect our mental health, but they also leave traces on our faces. And that makes us look older than we really are. I spoke from my own experiences. When I failed my study abroad and got depressed for over 5 years, I looked awful, miserable and older than now, the 30 year-old me. Being aware of yourself by living sympathetically and controlling your healthy weight is the only way to look younger and live blissfully more than ever.

These are pictures of me from 2013 and 2020.

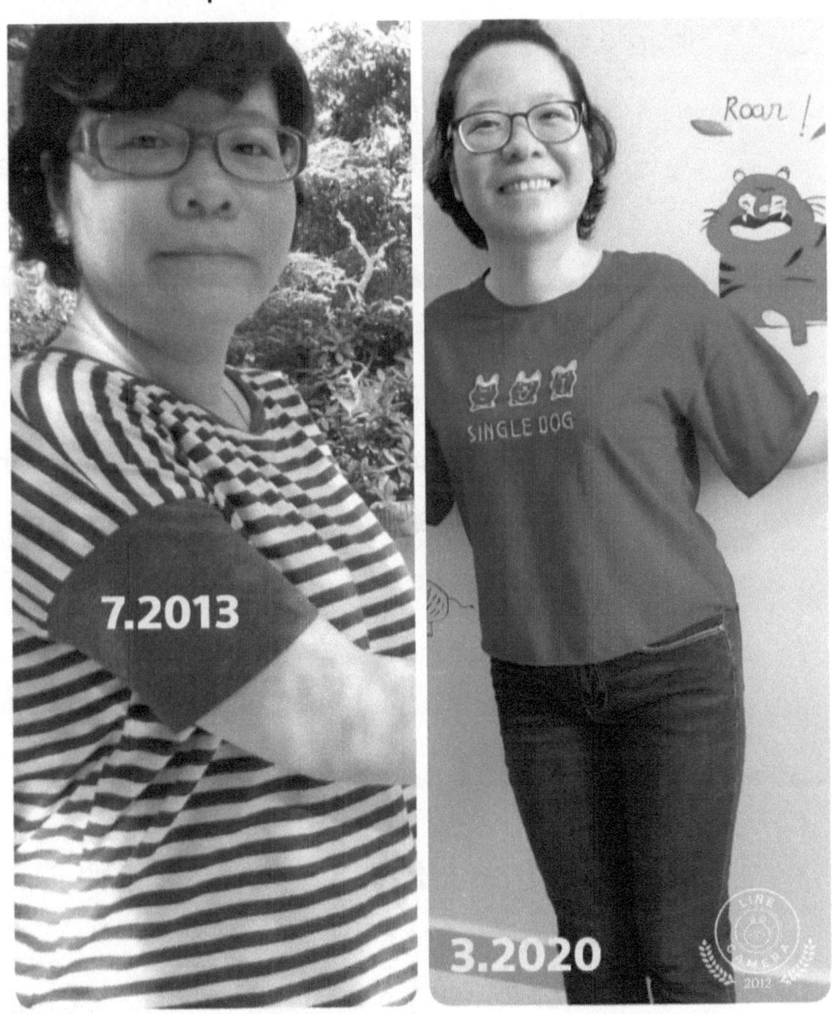

5. Try turmeric face mask 2-3 times a week

Ingredients:

- 3-4 pieces fresh turmeric
- About 1 litre of honey (wild honey or branded honey for the optimal result)

- 1 slice of lemon

Instruction:

- Peel, wash and then blend the turmeric well into the honey so as the quantity of honey is much more than blended turmeric (the honey covers the turmeric).
- Add some drops of lemon to this mixture.
- Pour it into a glass jar and leave it in the fridge for at least a month.

How to use:

- Wash your face before using it. Then, apply a thin coat of it on your face.
- After leaving it on your face for 30 minutes or so, wash it off with warm water, then rinse your face with cool water.

Tips: You'll notice how smooth your skin gets after performing this routine 2-3 times a week for several months.

This turmeric mask is sensitive to sunlight, so make sure to protect your skin properly by avoiding direct sunlight.

Chapter 2: Anti-aging by self-control

I suggest some healthy daily diets which keep you energized all day.

Some healthy recipes

1. Baked pork ribs

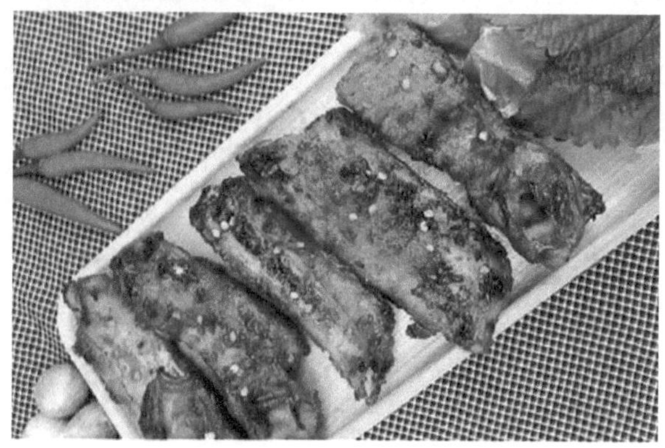

(daynauan.info.vn)

Ingredient:

- Pork ribs or pork cutlets ½ kg (4 cups)
- Lemon grass 2 sprigs
- Garlic 3 cloves
- Sugar ½ tsp
- Salt, chopped fresh chili (remove the seeds), soy sauce, and MSG to taste.

Instruction:

- Clean the pork ribs and chop them into pieces around 3cm (1.2 inches) wide. If you are using pork cutlets, chop them into pieces around 4cm (1.5-1.6 inches) wide.

- Mince the lemon grass and garlic, mix with half a teaspoon of sugar, salt, a little chopped chili and a dash of MSG.

- Pour soy sauce on them. Let the pork marinate in the mixture for 1 hour. They will taste good when you grill them.

- Bake until they become yellow brown. Don't let them burn.

2. Ground pork wrapped in cabbage soup

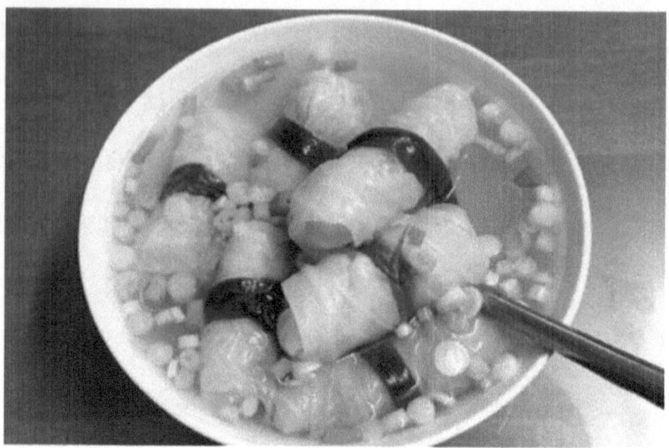

(nauzi.com)

Ingredient:

- Ground pork 1 cup (200g)

- Fresh shrimp 0.5 cup (100g)

- Cabbage 10 leaves

- 10 green onions, cilantro, salt, pepper, a dash of MSG or 1 teaspoon of pork stock powder, and sugar to taste.

Instruction:

- Clean pork and shrimp, ground them together with 2 cloves of gree onions. Then mix them well with a little sugar, half a teaspoon of salt, pepper.

- Separate cabbage and green onions to clean them. Blanch them for 15 seconds.

Fish them out of the boiling and drain them into colander. Slice cabbage a half. Remove the core in the end.

- 1 teaspoon of ground pork will be wrapped in each cabbage leaf. Then use 1 sprig of green onions to tie.

- After finishing, put all into boiling water. Seasoning the water by a dash of MSG or pork stock powder, or add any season mentioned above if you like. When it reaches the boiling point, remove any scums that float the top.

- Before serving, garnish with some minced green onions and a dash of cilantro.

3. Waxy pumpkin soup

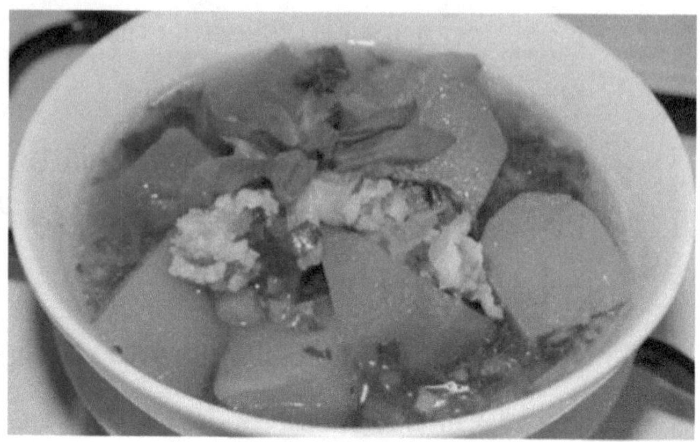

(daotaobeptruong.vn)

Ingredient:

- 1 new, fresh waxy pumpkin

- Lean meat 0.5 cup (100g)

- Shrimp 0.5 cup (100g)

- Green onions, salt, pepper, sugar, MSG to taste.

Instruction:

- Remove the green rind of the waxy pumpkin, clean it well. Remove its core.

- Cut pumpkin into pieces that are 5cm wide.

- Peel shrimps, clean them with salt.

- Chop meat, shrimps with green onions, mix them with salt, pepper, a dash of MSG, sugar. Mix them well. Leave it for 15 minutes.

- Put shrimps and meat into boiling water. Put waxy pumpkin into the same pot. Taste it. Pumpkin will taste good if it's not too soft.
- When it reaches boiling point, remove the bubbles that have floated to the top.
- Don't put the lid on the pot.
- Before serving, put some minced green onions and a dash of pepper on top.

4. Egg drop soup with tomato and seasoned seaweed

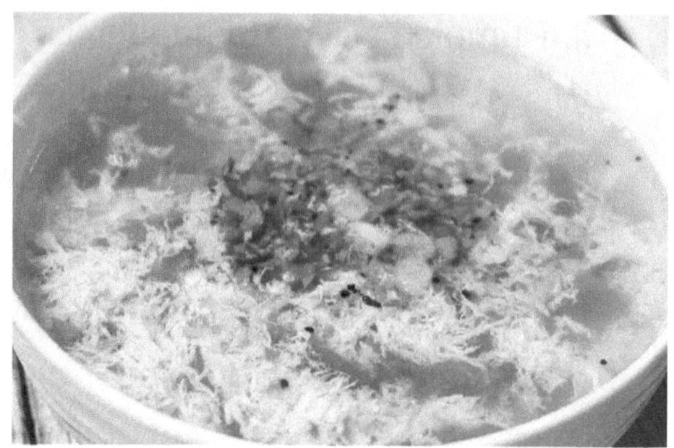

(thucthan.com)

Ingredient:

- Ripe tomatoes 4 medium-sized.

- 2 eggs + 1 tbsp water.

- Cooking oil 1 tbsp.

- Water 100ml (0.5 cup)

- Salt ½ tsp.

- A dash of MSG, fish sauce (optional)

- 1 pinch pepper.

- Sesame oil 1-2 tbsp.

- 1-3 packs of seasoned seaweed snack.

Instruction:

- Cut the tomatoes into small cubes.

- Crack the eggs into a bowl. Add 1 tablespoon of water to the eggs. Add a dash of MSG. Whisk until smooth.
- Stir fry tomatoes on med-high heat in a pot with a dash of MSG or a little of fish sauce (optional).
- Pour water into this pot and wait until it's boiling.
- When it reaches boiling point, turn heat down to low. Put the lid on loosely.
- When the water begins to boil again, uncover and slowly pour in the egg while swirling it around with a spoon.
- Season to taste it with salt, pepper and sesame oil.
- Turn off the heat. Add seasoned seaweed snack pieces into it.
- Before serving, sprinkle some pepper on.

5. Tofu stir-fry with ground pork

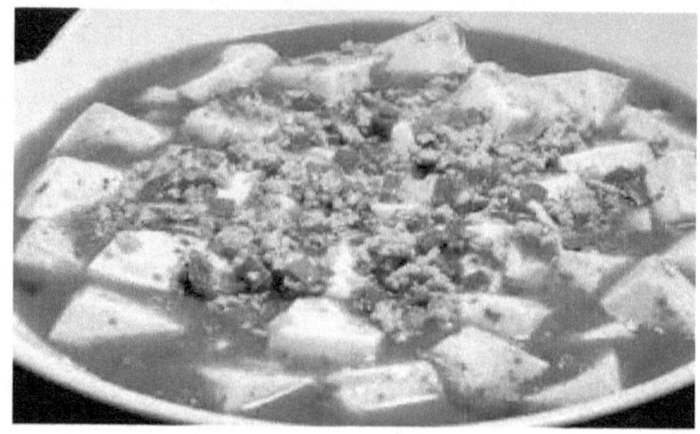

(baobacgiang.com.vn)

Ingredient:

- Oyster sauce: ½ tbsp

- Package firm tofu drained: 2 pieces

- Ground pork: 0.5lb (200g)

- Tomato: 2

- MSG: ½ tsp

- Sugar: ½ tsp

- Garlic: 1 glove

- Pepper, salt, minced shallot, green onion to taste.

Instruction:

- Mix ground pork with a dash of MSG, a dash of pepper, salt, minced shallot. Mince tomato. Cut tofu into equal pieces. Mince garlic.

- Put cooking oil in your pan. Wait until it's going to hot then pour garlic on it. Stir fry for a couple of seconds. Put minced tomato in it and keep stirring fry until tomato becomes a compound.

- Pour ground pork into that compound and stir fry quickly for 1 minute.

- Taste it then pour ½ a cup of water in it, stir fry roughly for 2 minutes. After that, pour tofu into it and stir fry gently. Taste them with 1 tsp of oyster sauce or so. Lighten heat until the sauce is syrupy. Turn off the heat. Ornate it with a dash of pepper, green onion.

Try aloe vera juice

According to Rick Hay, the superfoodist, aloe vera can help us reduce internal inflammation, eczema and rosacea thanks to its detoxifying, antimicrobial, and antiviral properties. We also should drink fruit juice with a ratio of juice to water of ¼ and ¾ respectively. This ratio will let you enjoy the taste without triggering insulin production, which is one of the leading causes of obesity. He suggested we should consider enjoying whole fruit and vegetables because they include fibre.

Tip 1: Eat everything you like in moderation

You will be fatter quicker than you think. Losing weight is not a phase, it just a habit you can train yourself into maintaining throughout your life. I try my best to keep a close eye to anything I eat. If it is suitable for me, it will suitable for everyone because I'm a lazy person who wants to foresee result first then I'll make a habit of it. According to scientific research, you can make one new habit in 21 days, I believed it and sometimes I made my new habit in 10 days, it works for me. The kind of things like a 10 days jogging challenge, drink 2l of water challenge in 30 days, etc. You should teach your body what to eat for your greatest benefit. And you'd adopt a belief that provides you with the greatest health so you are relaxed even while being productive.

Tip 2: Think optimistically, try to laugh as much as you can

That's the simplest method to lose weight I experienced myself for a long time. When I was fat, I used to be a hilarious but shy person. On my way to lose weight, I'm usually into my favorite thing: laughter. Yes, that it is. Try to take a real smile when you watch a rom-com, cartoon or maybe when doing chores in daily life. A big laugh can also work your belly muscles. Stress causes a build up of cortisol and adrenaline which can over your digestive system leading to flatulence and bloating. So please don't make stress stay by your side!

Tip 3: Drink enough water

You should drink water all day as formula: your weight x 0.04, is the water you need for a day to work well. People believed you should drink 2-2.5l of water each day. From my experience, 1.5l-2l of diluted lemon juice per day can make a significant difference. Not only it helps you lose weight, but it also makes your skin glow and feel smoother. And you will be release from constipation also. Dehydration is a leading cause of constipation. The digestive system needs plenty of water to keep food waste moving through it.

Drinking plenty of water and healthful juices can help relieve constipation in many cases. My recipe of diluted lemon juice is one of the most simple healthy drinks for you all who suffer from constipation. It contains 1-1.5l water with half a small lemon. Mix it well and you can drink all day long instead of drinking water. It worked well with me who had constipation issues for over 10 years. For that reason, it should work well for you. Anyway, the quantity of water depends on your activities, weather or maybe your stomach.

As part of my daily routine, I drink diluted lemon juice followed by some warm water everyday. I usually drink diluted lemon juice and warm water. Sometimes before going to bed, I will drink a cup of warm water with honey for a better night's sleep. Always keep your body hydrated when exercising. It is easy to become dehydrated and not even know it. I usually drink 1l of diluted lemon juice when working out. As you know, our bodies are comprised of 70% water:

Brain: 74.5%

Blood: 83%

Kidneys: 82.7%

Muscles: 75.6%

Bone: 22%

If you become dehydrated there is a 2% to 3% drop in your resting metabolic rate.

That's why too little water can cause the body to become weaker under tremendous strain. Drinking enough water brings dual benefits to your body for both mental and physical health. You flush toxins from your system and avoiding weight increase from empty snacking at the same time.

Another benefit to drinking plenty of water is that it keeps your muscles pumped and ready for action.

Tip 4: Losing weight but not losing your appetite

Enjoy your meals with close-knit people is a good way to control your weight too. I used to gain weight when I'm blue because I have to eat alone, far away with my parents and friends. But after I have meals with them everyday, I eat with joy and lose weight naturally.

The reason restrictive calorie diets usually don't work is because of our genetics. Cut back on food and our survival instinct thinks we are heading for a famine, causing our mind-body system to "stock up" and store fat.

An ongoing research shows that diet changes alone are ineffective in 97% of adults after five years. Diet with exercise is better, and only lifestyle change is truly effective.

Only eat when you need to

Each of your meals should be at least 4 hours apart. Try to chew slowly by counting 1 to 20 in your head. Try to stop eating when you feel nearly full or practicing Hara Hachi Bu's rule everyday until it becomes your habit. It helps you to control your weight loss progress and not feel tired throughout the day.

Tip 5: Keep a weight loss diary or note on your phone

If you're not sure you are keeping your weight on track or not, it helps you stay on track. I have a note on my phone in order to keep up with my progress. After waking up while I have an empty stomach, I measure my body (chest, belly, butt and weight index). I check those indexes every month for acknowledge my improvement. So I won't be distracted from meeting my goal.

Keep in mind that diet, stress or inflammation are often at the root of enzyme deficiencies, and a quick and easy supplement might not always be the best answer. "the biggest factor that affects poor digestion is going to be eating too fast, eating too big of a meal, and being stressed out while you do it," said Dr.Tim Gerstmar, a seattle-based naturopathic doctor and a digestive health and autoimmune specialist.

Chapter 3: How could I lose nearly 28 pounds without a trainer within 7 months?

Losing weight progress needs three elements: exercises, diet, and attitude. I'm not a professional trainer and this is not my area of expertise, I just tried many ways to lose weight and keep anti-aging as long as I can for many years. I know this one thing: if you find many ways to change yourself as an active way a little bit every single day, to enhance your health, or maybe to feel good, you can be happier day by day. Losing weight is the best way to cure disease and look pretty without surgery. If I, a lazy like sloth can do it, then I believe everyone who has willpower can do it also. These interesting tips below are the best things you can do for your mental and physical well-being.

I used to be naturally lean, but as time went on, I got fatter every year. At its worst, my peak weight was 143.3lbs (65kg).

I hit the gym 2 year ago from March 2018 until the end of this year. After losing nearly 28 pounds (from 143.3pounds to 116 pounds (53kg) with a height of 4'12 (152cm)), I stopped losing weight. It was a problem for a long time. After I found that my interest in the gym was the main factor in my weight, I started doing cardio on the Youtube channel at home taught by Susana Yabar. To me, she is a star, a mentor even though I'd never met her in real life. Her cardio workouts helped me learn more about my body. If you get a weight loss plateau, you can try another solution to reach your ideal, healthy weight. The key here is to eat more and exercise more or eat less to do less. The outtake must always be moderately bigger than the intake.

Tip 1: Eat fruits and vegetables like main meals at least once a day

The way that you exercise every day is not important to the way you eat. For me, at least I eat the fruit in 1 meal entirely. And one crucial thing to remember that making fruit a meal must include traffic light color. That's mean it must have green, red, yellow color fruit such as cucumber, tomato, papaya, banana, bell pepper, etc..

Eat good carbs instead of bad carbs. You can choose sweet potatoes, red rice, some kinds of beans like peanuts, green beans or so on you can find in the market. Anyway, an ideal meal should contain food from the soil and sea. You know what I mean. Food from the soil like fruits, vegetables, etc. And foods from the sea are fish, seaweed, etc.

Tip 2: Let water waken you up every morning

When I'm still sleepy even though I wake up every morning, I drink a cup of warm water (300ml-500ml) then lay back in my bed for 30 minutes. Then a new day starts from there. A study[3] published in 2003 showed that drinking warm water in the morning can help increasing metabolism and weight loss. *"about 40% of the thermogenic effect originated from warming the water from 22 to 37 °C. In men, lipids mainly fueled the increase in metabolic rate. In contrast, in women carbohydrates were mainly used as the energy source"*.

---

[3] Boschmann M, Steiniger J, Hille U, Tank J, Adams F, Sharma AM, Klaus S, Luft FC, Jordan J. Water-induced themogenesis. https://www.ncbi.nlm.nih.gov/pubmed/14671205

Tip 3: Approach positively and enjoy yourself

Keep an eye on your weight but don't obsess over it every day. If it's necessary, measure your weight and body index once a month to know how you have improved or need to exercise more. When doing exercises every day, you don't need to work as long as you can but try to sweat as much as possible even if you only have 15 minutes a day working out. I installed a heart rate app for tracking my workouts at home. When you work out enough to make your heart rate higher than average and you sweat a lot, that means your stubborn body fat is being worked away. When we engage in exercise, our body adjusts to the new level. If we then cut back slightly, even a small decline in the number of calories burned will make it more difficult to lose weight. One more essential thing you should remember is your fat-burning heart rate is at about 70% of your maximum heart rate. For example, my burning heart rate is 130bpm-160bpm when working out and 70bpm-90bpm for resting. Too much and too little is not good. The right way is the optimal thing.

Tip 4: Listen to your body

We tend to eat everything we can reach with terrific speed after going home exhausted. I was an avid foodie who ate everything I could get my hands on. One day, I read about the Japanese Hara Hachi Bu's rule and how the Okinawan people can live over 100 years just by following this ordinary rule. Besides healthy food and the scientific way of living, they practice Hara Hachi Bu every day until it becomes one of their habits. In Japanese language, Hara Hachi Bu means your belly's 8 out of 10. So this magical spell means you shouldn't eat more when you feel a bit full even if there is enough room for another bite.

Just eat 80% of what your belly can bear or maybe eat until you don't feel hungry anymore. As I said, eat in moderation. When you eat, your stomach takes 20 minutes signal to your brain it's full. One crucial thing you should do to control your eating speed is to eat slowly and joyfully. Focus on your meal. Count to 20 in your mind while grabbing a bite and wait.

Your stomach feels at ease after a meal, not stressed. You are not breathing hard because you ate all that you could. It takes within one week or more to make your stomach get used to eating less. I noticed I can handle it tactfully after 2 weeks of practicing. Most of us are used to overeating which is past satiation and which keeps weight on. According to a registered dietician, Susan Dopart[4], *once we begin to feel any stomach pressure, we are at the "80 percent full" stage.*

Anyway, all healthy food, homemade food which suit you deserve your enjoyment during eating. You should eat only when you feel hungry. And eat with love of nature and you will feel eager at every meal.

We should eat to live but in my opinion, we should only eat about 70% of our whole energy we need per day.

Controlling your weight is the way to show how strong your mind is. Failure to control your weight does not mean you're weak but it shows you're

4 Irene Rubaum-Keller. Hara Hachi Bu: eat until you are 80% full. 09/21/2011.
https://www.huffpost.com/entry/not-overeating_b_969910

incapable of loving yourself as much as you deserve. You are the owner of your mind.

Tip 5: Manage cravings

Remember to take a deep breath to overcome the strong desire to eat, and think about why you shouldn't eat it for a moment. For example, it works like preventing yourself from smoking. You relax your mind and keep your body engaged until the desire passes out. You need to allow the longing at present and wait until it stops. You'll see how it works day by day. As for me, every time I get the desire to eat junk food, I lie down and breathe using my stomach for a while. When I relax my mind and concentrate solely on my breathing, I can sense how it works better. When doing so, I control my desire to eat junk food and I burn belly fat in the process. After doing this regularly, I noticed it helped my body and mind connect and my belly quickly got noticeably smaller. If you're having trouble with this breathing exercise, try slowly taking a small sip of water until you feel better.

Chapter 4: Small habits often lead to big changes.

1. What should I do after meal?

After meals, I usually stand or walk around my room for at least 25 minutes. It helps digest your meal without putting pressure on your stomach. In this period time, you can do anything you want providing you keep yourself standing with a straight back. I don't drink while standing to allow my stomach time to digest properly. Some proof from scientific studies suggests we should drink water 30 minutes to 1 hour after a meal in order to absorb nutrition.

Your bad feelings are your inner enemy

Every time you feel like you're bursting with anger, take note of why you feel that right away. But if you are a lazy person like me, you can do it simply by imagining while belly breathing. Try to evoke a bad feeling in your mind and visualize how it does to your body if it wins. What you can do to overcome it or maybe, for best result, make it never happens to you. I usually use my trick that bad feeling is like a joke or a ball I can play with it all day to control my mind. Why should we allow it to make us feel bad or revoke our energy?

You may soak in positive emotions such as gratitude, love, sympathy, etc. Wrap yourself up with emotions to get you motivated to stop stress and gain weight. This exercise will be regularly used to provide a healthy armor for difficult emotions. Think of the person, place or thing that activates the emotion, and feel and visualize as you breathe. Make it real in your mind and body to express the emotion as you breathe. Even simply continue saying a word in your mind will crop up the response you're searching for. Recalling one of the most happiest memory, for example, can be the only trigger you need to evoke the feeling. Stick with it while you practice deep breathing, keeping your attention on the word or accident. You'll see how you get better. Or you should blank your mind while doing belly breathing. Think nothing and just keep focus on flow of breath goes in and out of your belly. Count you breath by seconds if you like.

"stretch and repeat the belly breathing pattern until you feel calm and peaceful. Through

your breathing, you will have signaled to yourself that you are in a safe environment and that you accepted (and thus respected) any of your emotions. You will be communicating with your inner self your desire to accept these emotions. You may notice that your shoulders and neck become more relaxed as you continue.

Moreover, you will also have disconnected some of your eating triggers during this process. Most people will notice a feeling of lightness and feeling better overall. Another positive result is you free the energy you had used to hold onto or suppress your stored emotions. You will now naturally feel much finer. Practicing belly deep breathing keeps your blood chemistry always be in the optimal range", wrote Thomas Goode[5], a doctor of naturopathy.

2. Go number two regularly, it's the key

Go number two every day if you can or 2 days once. I used to suffer constipation when I was a young age but after trying to lose weight, I found a diet rich in fruits solved my problem with double

---

[5] Thomas Goode,ND. The holistic guide to weightloss, anti-aging and fat prevention. 2005

benefits with keeping fit and smooth skin. Also keeping my stomach comfortable with ease. Fruit maniac grew on me every day. Try not to eat fruit rich in sugar like mangosteen but if you eat in moderation (fist-size), you'll find it can help you reduce your cravings.

3. Try donating your blood once every 4 months

How does this little thing help in losing weight? Not only does it make your skin smoother but it also strengthens your metabolism. Besides, this act can reduce harmful iron deficiency and the risk of developing cancer would also be decreased. Furthermore, your liver remains strong thanks to your blood donation to other people. So donating your blood is the give and take gift.

4. Try not to get mad over one time a week

Not only your anger leaves tracks on your face, but also it keeps your metabolism doesn't work well and most of all, it distracts you from your goal of losing weight healthily. If you get yourself down, you send a negative signal to your cells which takes away health and happiness from you.

5. Don't afraid to change your body

Since I was a university student, I had surgery done in my belly and there are still scars there until now. And I always felt tired when climbing upstairs even though it had only two flights. My belly grew bigger every day until the year before last (2018) when I looked at myself in the mirror and was wondering why I didn't do anything to get out of this case: bring an awkward person who has-to difficultly move anywhere. Hence I made up my mind and here I am (a self-proud person who is confident and happy). Changing my body index is the lifelong present I reward myself and so do you. It's a grant with effort and patience day by day. *"to be thin does not mean to be loved. Everyone has a certain healthy weight. You just need to identify your natural weight to keep you feel healthier. You deserve to be loved no matter what you look like or how much you weigh"*, said Thomas Goode[6], a naturopathic doctor.

---

[6] Thomas Goode,ND. The holistic guide to weightloss, anti-aging and fat prevention. 2005

6. Simple is the best

Nobody can pursue a trick diet long term because it's too hard to follow and be disciplined. So keep your diet as simple as possible is the best way to lose weight without any pressure. You can choose to eat any healthy foods you like. Keep foods rich in sugar at bay and have fun while eating. Do some light or intense exercise either every day to sweat. They are two main ways of natural detox for your mental and physical health.

However, it's annoying to measure everything you eat by calories. You should use your fist to measure your food to roughly get the correct food portion. This small trick works by quantifying them so you don't eat too much.

Chapter 5: Workouts at the gym and home.

Warming up - Do at your own pace

If you want to shed some unwanted pounds and to increase your fitness level regardless of age, you should do some moderate exercises at least 5-6 times per week to achieve optimal results. High-intensity interval training exercises or some professional exercises have been chosen for you, because these will get you the best fitness results in the shortest amount of time. But, they are hard for beginners, so you must follow at your own pace to decide what is suitable for you. No one knows you better than yourself, right?

Before working out at home or gym, I spend 5-10 minutes warming up my body.

1. Standing ankle rotation

-   Point your left toe to the ground

-   Rotate your ankles for 30 seconds in a clockwise direction then repeat for further 30 seconds in counterclockwise.

-   Repeat this action for the right toe.

2. Wrist circle

-   Grab your hands together.

- Rotate in clockwise for 30 seconds and then for further 30 seconds in a counterclockwise rotation.

3. Shoulder circle

- Move your arms forward to make a large circle as you can for 20 seconds.
- Then repeat backward for 20 seconds.

4. Alternating knee hug

- Stand upright while your left knee up to your chest, grab it for 10 seconds.
- Then repeat with the right knee for another 10 seconds.

5. Knee rotation

- Put your hands on your knees.
- Rotate your knees in the clockwise direction for 20 seconds, then reverse for another 20 seconds.

6. Side bends

- Stand with feet shoulder-width apart, grab your right hip with your right hand.
- Engage your core and bend at your waist, bringing your upper body to the right toward the floor.

- Standing straight, back to start position and repeat with the left side.
7. Jumping jacks
- Stand with your feet together and your arms against your sides.
- Hop and separate your feet to nearly shoulder-width apart while bringing your arms fully above your head (clapping if you like).
- Hop again while bringing your feet and arms back into the initial position.

Workouts at the gym

Aside from dieting, choosing enjoyable exercise is the most important part. When you enjoy working out you're more likely to stick with it. At the first time when I went to the gym where I used to call the giant robust world, for being a 143.3lbs (65kg) weight-person with the height of nearly 5ft (152cm), I found it tough doing exercises at the gym but it got easier as time goes by. Youtube is a tool you can use when you need to see how something is done properly. However, in my little book, I can tell you about my experiences of working out at the gym and at home. So I will focus on the tips, forms and some principles you should remember.

Treadmill

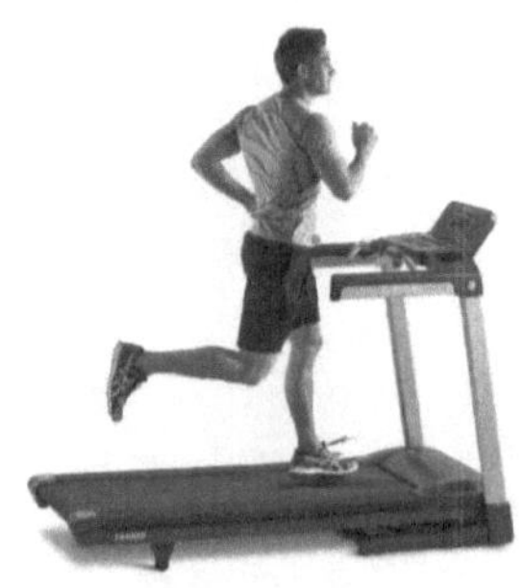

(lifespan fitness)

I started by jogging on a treadmill from 15 minutes to 30 minutes in the first week to keep track of my weight. A simple rule to remember is to keep focusing on distance, not your speed. Then I ate cucumbers and tomatoes instead of desserts for almost 3 main meals to lose weight. Cucumbers were additional food in the 3 main meals. During the second week, I combined a treadmill and stationary bike to let my body work faster. After being accustomed to them, I tried some more new interesting exercises that the gym had which I will show you below. For a good start, if you are quite unfamiliar with working out at the gym, you can go slowly and then increase the number of workouts in a week. For example, for the first week, you could do 3 days and in week 4, you could do 5 days. In case you just need its atmosphere for moving your body, you may try cardio (mostly exercises without dumbbells I will write below) at the gym. Do them at your own pace and then you'll see. Cardio can help you lose weight faster also.

When I go to the gym, I usually spend around 15 minutes per set, and I do 2 or 3 sets on the treadmill. I also do leg raises, and weight-related workouts depending on my mood that day. If I work on my legs too much today, then I will work on my chest tomorrow, and so on. You should focus on your body state and make schedule yourself based on your own needs.

Stationary bike

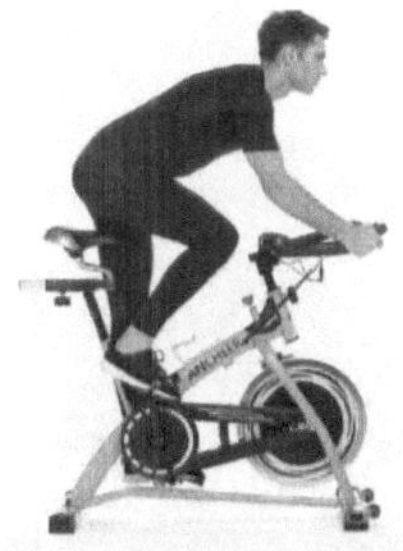

(newegg.com)

Before starting any more intense workout at the gym, I tried riding a stationary bike for at least 5 minutes to warm up my body. Instead of sitting on the seat of the bike, I stood to pedal as much as I could until I was sweating. You should warm up carefully before doing any weightlifting to avoid strain.

Seated cable low row (middle back muscles)

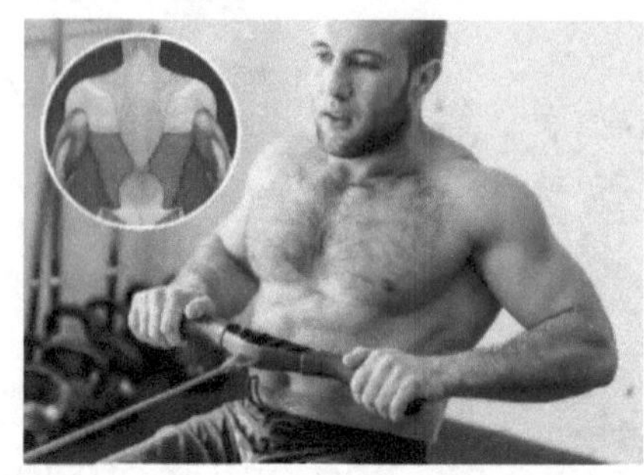

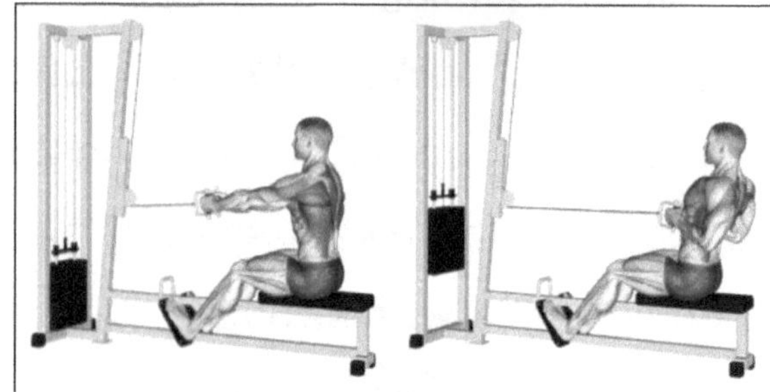

(brightside)

(apexcontestprep.com)

- Keep your back upright.
- Pull the handle bar slightly to your chest and hold it for a few seconds.
- Back to the initial position.

Lat pulldown (back)

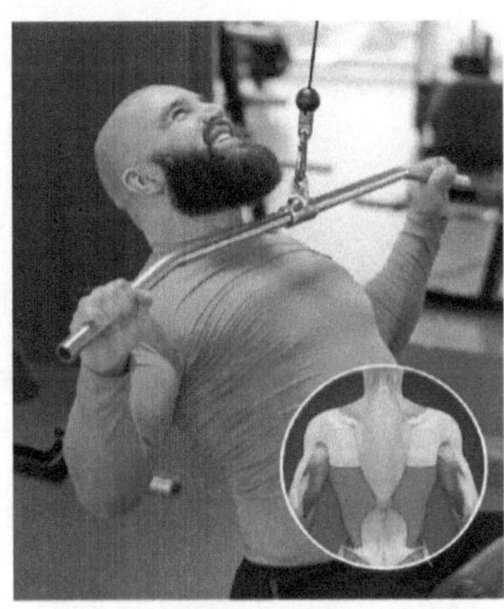

(brightside)

- If you are a male, your hands should be placed wider than a shoulder-width (in a wide grip). And if you are a female, your hands should be placed around shoulder-width.
- Your hands should be straight, and the bar should be over your head.
- When pulling it down, it should touch lightly to your chest.

Leg press (legs, thighs, glutes)

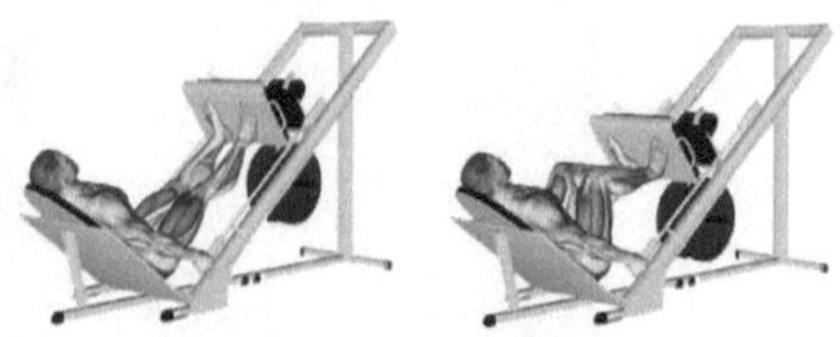

(thethaothientruong.vn)

By placing your feet differently, you can concentrate on the muscles you want.

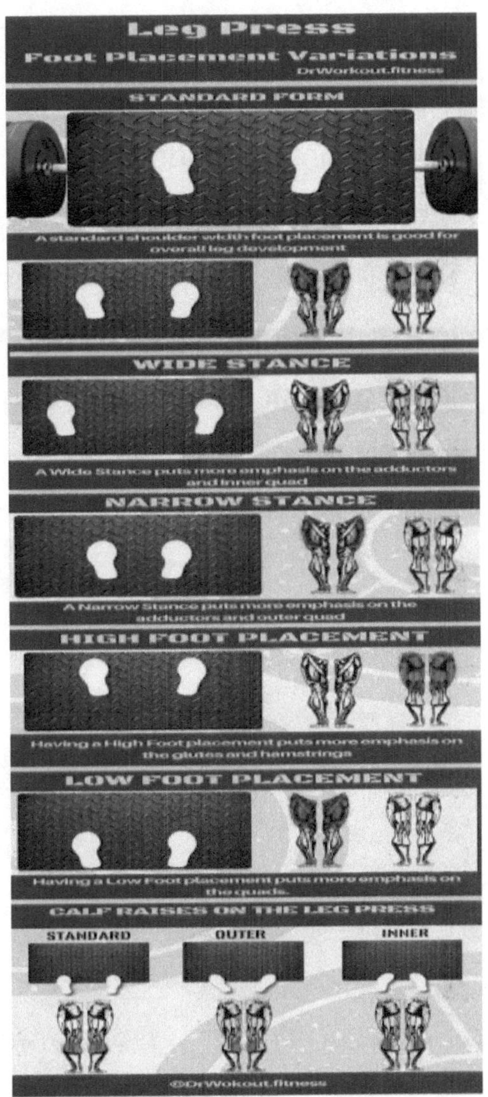

(drworkout.fitness)

- When your knees are at 90 degree angle,
  make sure they don't touch your chest. If
  they touch your chest, you may hurt your
  back later.
- Press the footplate up and straighten your
  legs (but not lock your legs, keep them
  slightly bent).

A single-arm bent-over row (good for your lats, traps, rear deltoids, and triceps.)

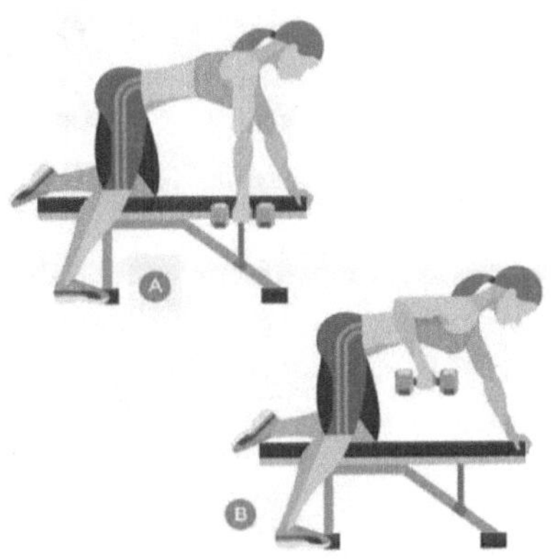

(women's health)

- You should not rotate or swing with your back, try to keep it still while lifting weight.
- Hold your upper body straight and still for the optimal result.
- You can start with 8-10 pounds (4-5kg) dumbbell.

Tricep extension (arm, back, chest)

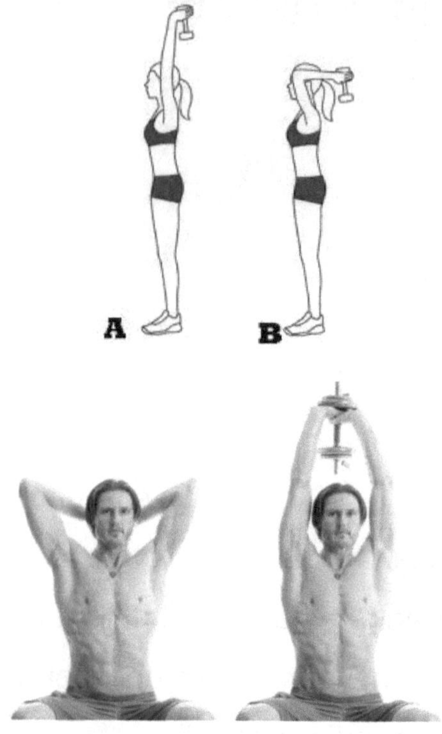

(pinterest.com)

(gaspari nutrition)

- Try to keep your elbows still while doing this exercise.

- Hold the dumbbell for a beat when you lift it over your head.

- Keep focus on your form (dumbbell holding way) and breathing speed, not your lifting speed.

Lunges (hip, thighs)

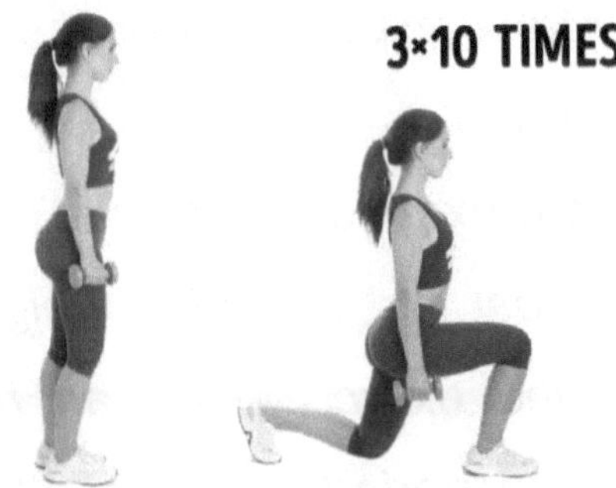

(© depositphotos.com)

- Bend your knee to 90 degree angle while stepping forward. Try not to let your other knee touch the ground, it will destroy the benefit of this exercise.

- You should feel extended in your lower body (especially the thighs and butt).

- You can hold dumbbell or not, it's up to you.

Tip: combining both cardio and weightlifting alternatively from time to time is a good way to keep your heart strong and build your muscles altogether.

How long should we do exercise?

Many experts suggest we should work out for 30 minutes [7]per day. 60 overweight Danish men *"who exercised for 30 minutes a day for three months lost just as much weight and body fat as those who exercised for an hour a day for the same time period"*. On the other hand, after you have lost a certain amount of weight, you will have to increase your training in order to see more weight loss.

Tiffany Mccoy[8], a well known personal trainer, she applied 30 minutes-over 1 hour each time and 'two-a-days' technique to reach her ideal goal weight. (for losing over 100lbs within 8 months) by increasing calorie burn. As far as I know, this is a good way to help upgrade your intensive training without putting much pressure on your muscles. For me, I cut down training time ups to each day's schedule. For instance, if I have more free time in day, I'll do exercise for 30 minutes twice a day. If I just get a few minutes at

---

[7] Live Science Staff. 2012.
https://www.livescience.com/22646-exercise-weight-loss.html

[8] Tiffany Mccoy. 100lbs.later. "How I lost over 100lbs.in 8 months and How YOU Can Do It Too!. 2015

interval, I like to work out for about 10 minutes and do so 3 times a day. Or I'll work out "round the clock" with small exercise each time. Anyway, the workout duration depends on your schedule so everyone has different times they like to work out. If you exceed your ideal body weight by 100lbs or more, you'll need to extend your training time by 30 minutes or more and consistently exercise twice a day. A great quote in her book says: if they (gymers) can do it, she can do it. In my case, I modified it to: if Tiffany (who used to be 250lbs weight) could do it, we can do it too. All you need is the love you invest in yourself. Nothing compares to how great you feel when you are on the right track of healthier you.

Workouts at home.

You should do these exercises below at home when you're familiar with doing workouts at the gym or maybe when you are trying to increase your fat-burning process. I did these things when I'd gotten to nearly 53kg or 116lbs (my height is 152cm or nearly 4ft12in) to stop putting too much pressure on my heart. You can make an attempt doing each muscle separately in a sequence or work on one muscle group at a time. For example, day 1 for butt, day 2 for the belly, day 3 for chest, day 5 for legs, day 6 for arms, off at day 7 and so on. Or do chest, abs, butt workout every day for 30 minutes, it depends on your fitness level. I prefer working out at home rather than in the gym because of the flexibility and weather. I'm the kind of person who is always eager to try new thing so I love to make my daily workout a little harder from time to time. In days when I am tired or blue, I like working out at home with random workouts from this list below.

1 minute or so jog on the spot for warming up

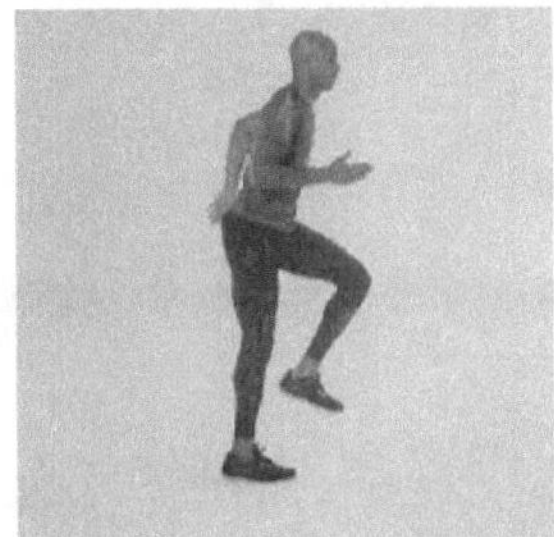 (skimble.com) 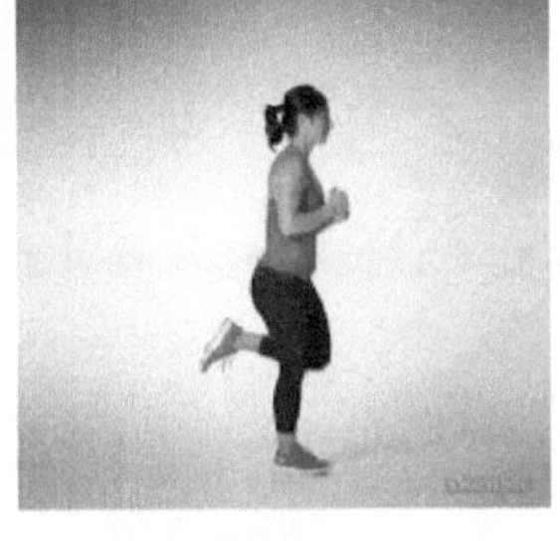

Lift your feet off the floor as fast as you can

Backward walking (good for body balance, memorable skill)

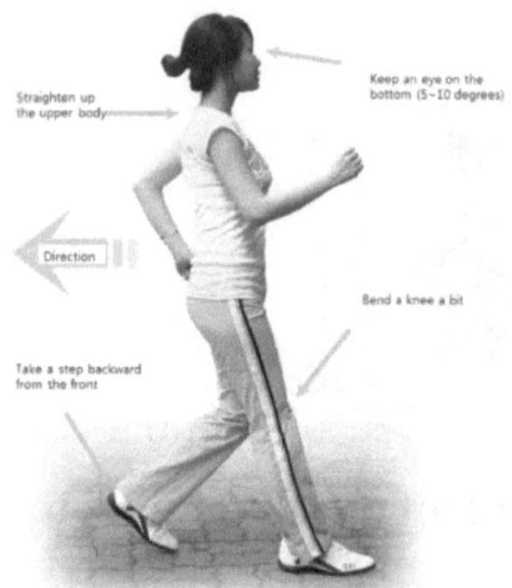

(wooriduhospital.wordpress.com)

- While increasing your pace, take shorter steps rather than longer ones. By doing this, you'll burn more calories. If it's raining outside, do this in your home. Simply crank up the music and enjoy!
- I usually do this small exercise while waiting for elevator.

1-minute knee raise for warming up (legs)

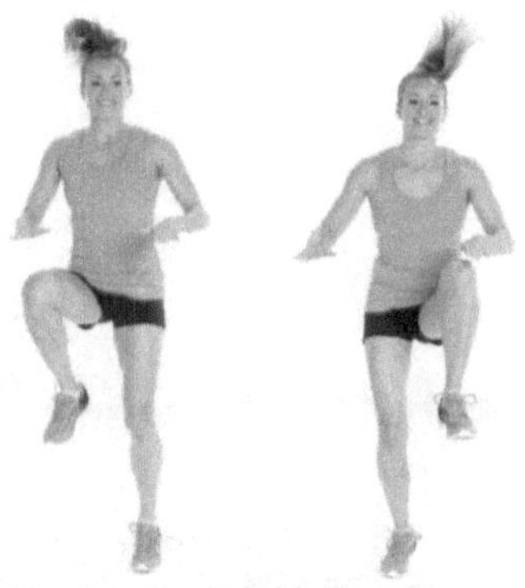

(popsugar)

- Put your hands (palms down) at the height between chest and waist. When you lift your legs, try to touch your knees with your hands.
- Keep breathing normally. You may start at slow pace then increase gradually.
- This position is like 'high jogging on the spot'

The cobra pose (chest)

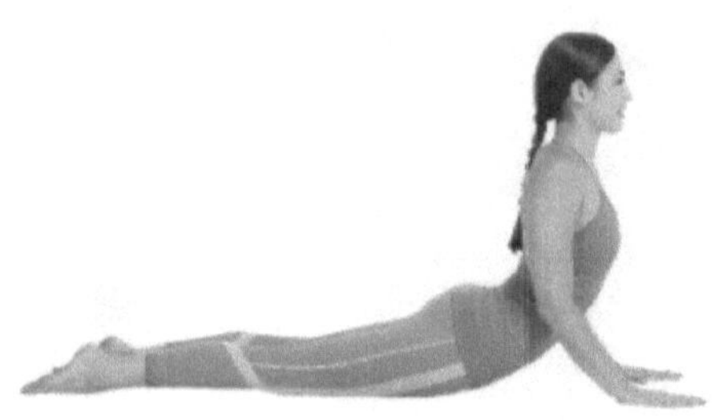

(yoga journal)

- Keep your neck straight, look forward. Relax, like you're looking up watching the sea in front of your eyes.
- You should feel a little extended on your belly while lifting your uppper body. Keep focus on your breath, and form.
- This pose is like the push up position with your chest and face down close to the floor and your arms supporting all your body to lift up.
- If you overdo it by using with sudden hard jerks, it'll hurt your back or neck.

A dumbbell floor press (chest)

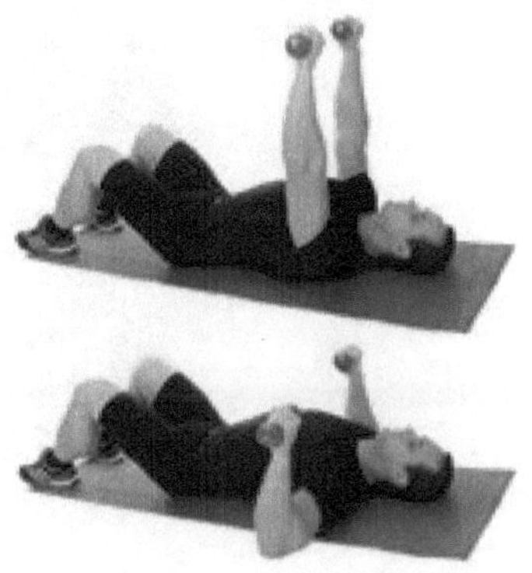

(pinterest)

- Keep your arms tight and straight (without locking your arms). When you put the dumbbells down, the dumbbells will be in the line with your nipples.
- Breathe in when lowering, breathe out when lifting.

Mountain climb (good for butt and belly)

x 8

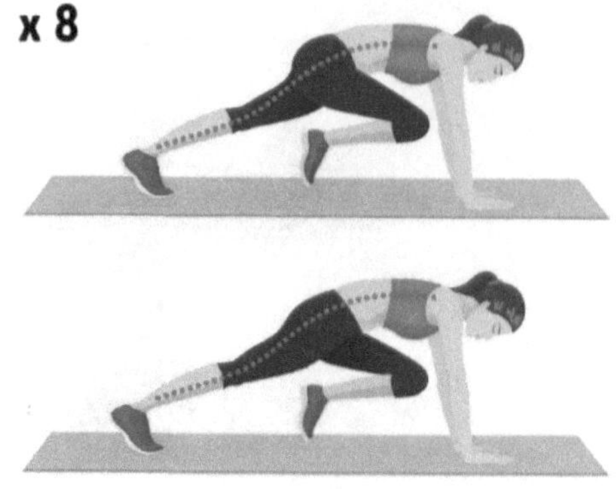

(brightside)

-   Your back should be straight or slightly bent, it must be in a natural position.
-   The key here is trying to touch your knees to your chest and your arms are under your shoulders.

Forearm plank (abs, glutes, arms)

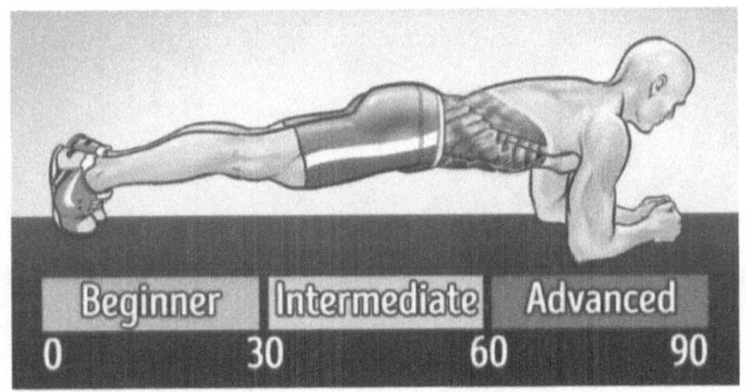

(brightside.me)

- Squeeze your belly, try to keep it aligned with your legs.
- Keep your neck straight by looking about 10 cm (4 inch) from your hands.
- Make sure you don't bend your lower back.

When you feel your body is shivering, try to hold the position for 15 seconds longer. You can do it.

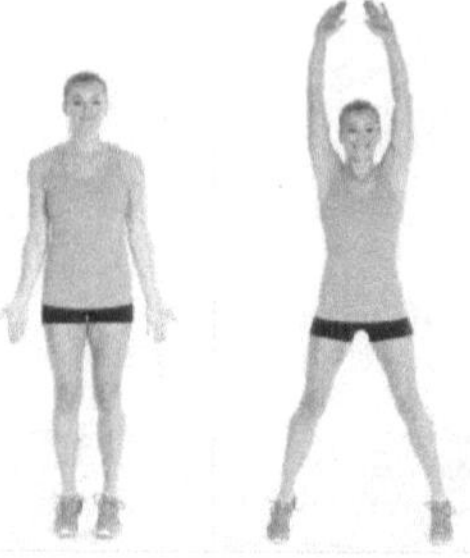

Jumping jack for full-body burning fat

(popsugar)

- Slightly jump off the floor. It works based on your speed, not the height.
- Your knees should face outwardly slightly. (like they should make a letter "v" together).

Bodyweight squat (for pretty butt)

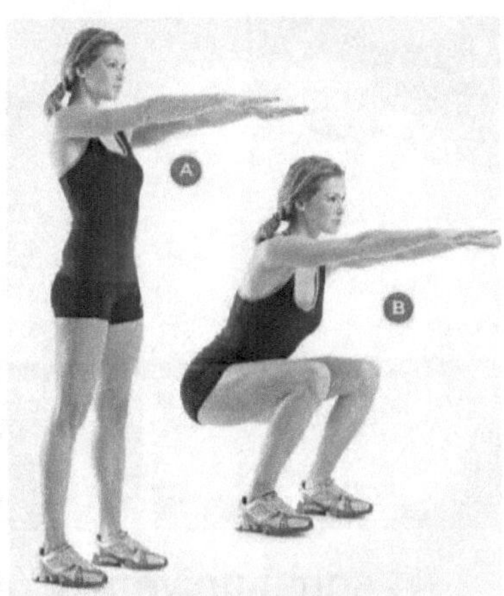

(Oprah.com)

- Like sitting on the invisible chair, you put 70% of your weight (when sitting down) on the heel of your feet, 30% left on your toes.

- Keep your back straight without putting any pressure on your back or it will hurt while doing the squat position. You should keep your eyes focused forward.

- This pose is like you're leaning over the rear ends sticking up to the people behind you.

Caution:

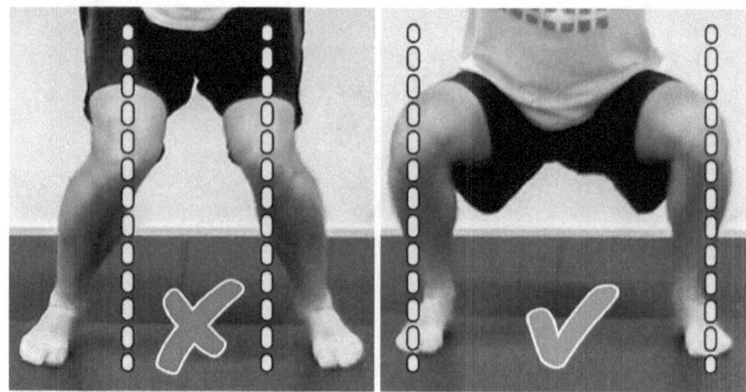

(© squat university / twitter)

Spread your legs like a standard "v" letter.

Jumping squat helps to lift your butt and burning body fat

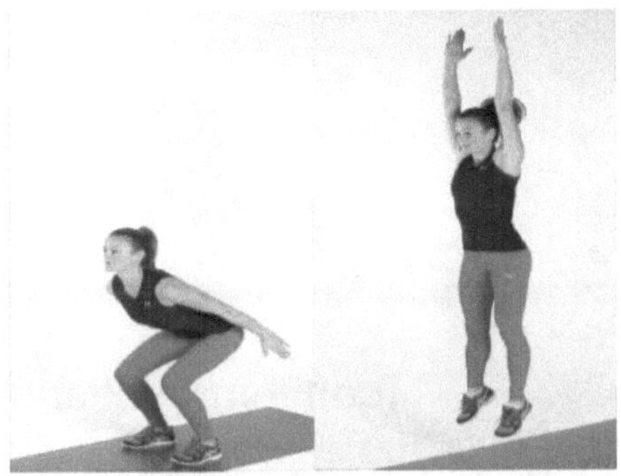

(popsugar)

- Keep your back straight, your eyes look forward.
- Breathe normally.

Reverse lunges (lower body)

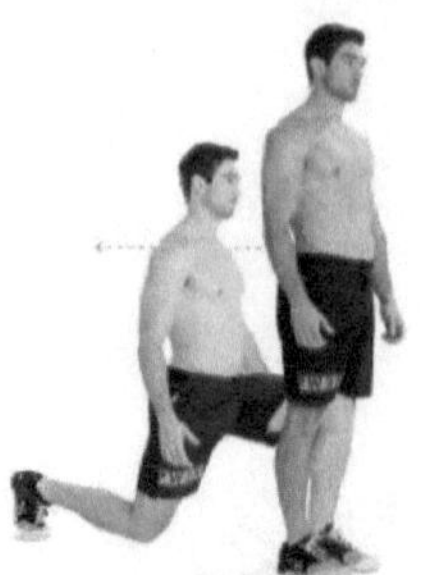

(coachmag.co.uk)

- Don't touch your knee to the ground, keep it 90 degrees to your body.
- Keep your chest up and your eyes ahead.

Curtsy lunge (thighs, glutes)

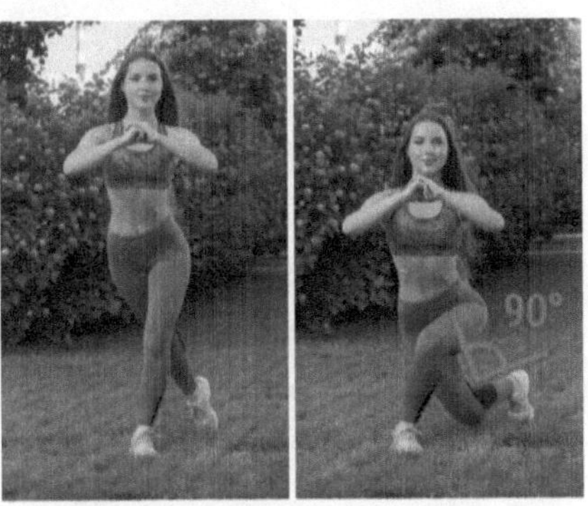

(© depositphotos.com)

Don't let your knee touch the ground. You should feel a little extended at your thighs.

Wall sit (lower body)

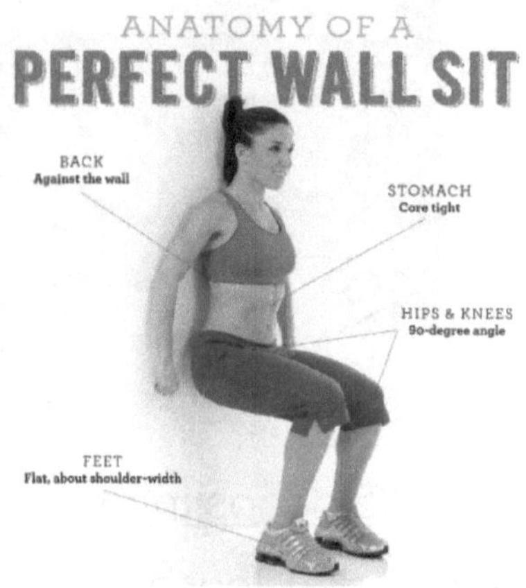

(ufcgym.com.vn)

- Start by standing hip-width legs apart. Then slowly sit down on the invisible chair.

- Keep your knees 90 degrees with the wall.

- Your back and neck should be close to the wall. Always make sure to keep your chest up and eyes looking straight ahead.

Wall legs up (good for the belly, butt, blood circulation, digestion, regardless fitness level)

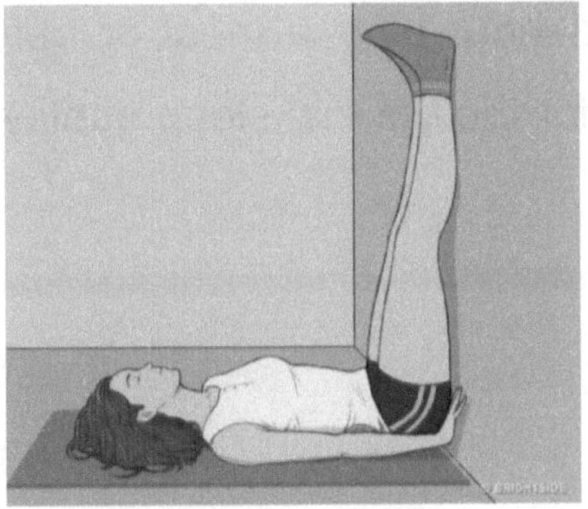

(brightside)

- Lying down, lift your legs and stretch them along the wall. Put your hands by your side.

- Your butt should be attached to the wall or at most 5 cm (nearly 2 inches) separate from the wall.

- Stay in this position for 10-15 minutes or 5 minutes each time, and do this 2-3 times.

- During this pose, if you feel your legs aching, you can slowly put them on the ground (by putting your legs against the wall) and then turn your body to the side. Take a short break for 20 to 30 seconds and then keep going until you finish.

-   This position is good for relaxing your whole body mentally and physically. You can do it 1 hour after a meal or before going to bed for the optimal sleep quality.

Heel touch (good for obliques)

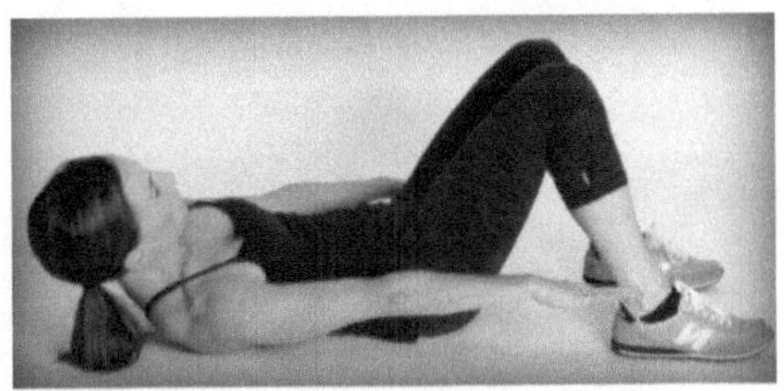

(fueled physique)

- Bend your knees, keep your feet on the ground.
- Move your upper body side to side, try to touch your ankles with your hands if possible.
- You should keep your head on a natural position to avoid hurting it.
- Keep focusing on your movement, not your speed.

Leg raise (legs, butt, core)

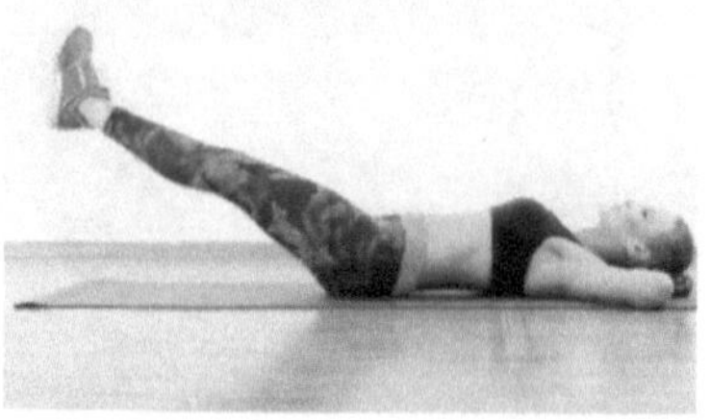

(cathe.com)

- Lie on your back, put your legs together and lift them up and down (keep them straight).
- Lift them up to 45 degrees or more, then slowly lower them back to the ground. Repeat.

Toe walking (calves)

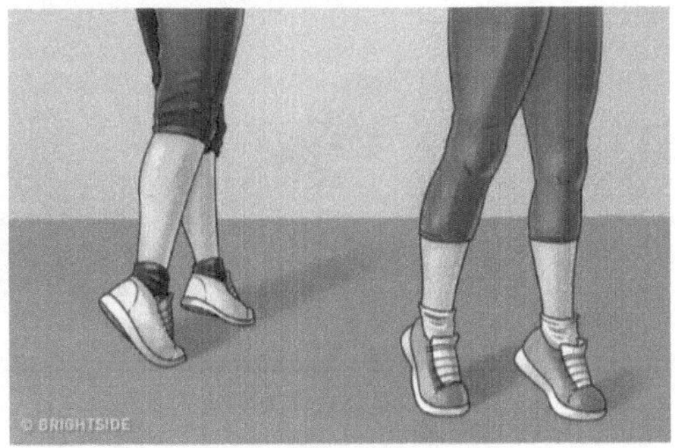

(brightside)

- This is one of the most simplest exercise I've ever known: walk on your toes until you feel tired. Do it whenever you want, with no limited time.

- Imagine you are walking like a ballerina.

Hip bridge (lower body)

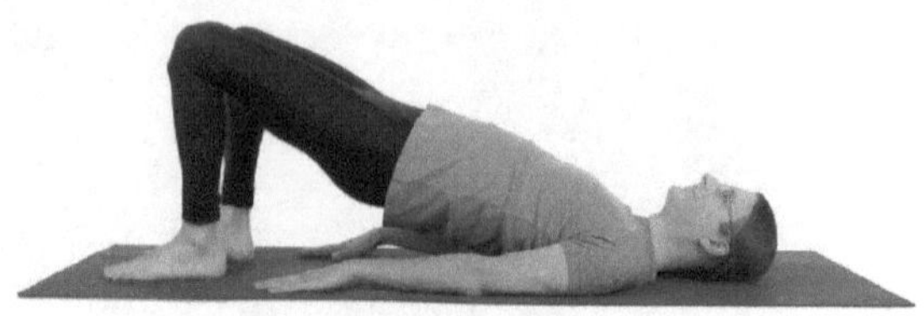

(summer season)

- Lay on the ground and bend your knees. While keeping your shoulders and feet on the floor, lift your belly until they are on a straight line with your shoulders and knees.
- Squeeze your butt while holding this position for 5-10 seconds.
- Lower down your belly, trying not to touch the ground with your butt.

Glute march (lower body)

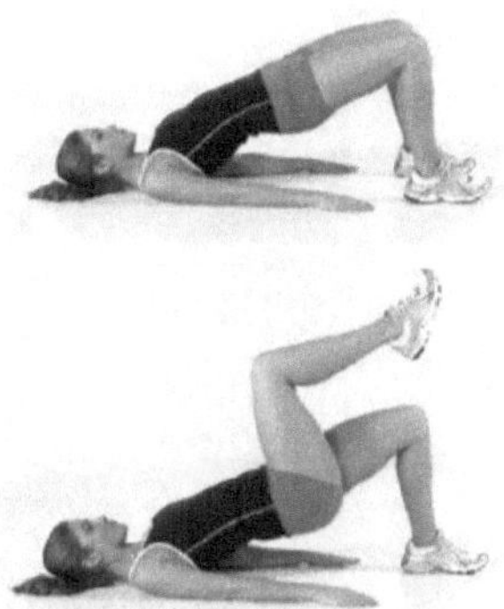

(bretcontreras.com)

- Do as the same position with hip bridge but you lift one leg toward your breast until your hip is 90 degree angle while keep the other leg on the floor.
- How it works depending on your form, not your speed.
- When lowering it down, try to keep your knee off the floor the other leg is still 90 degree angle.

Donkey kick (glutes)

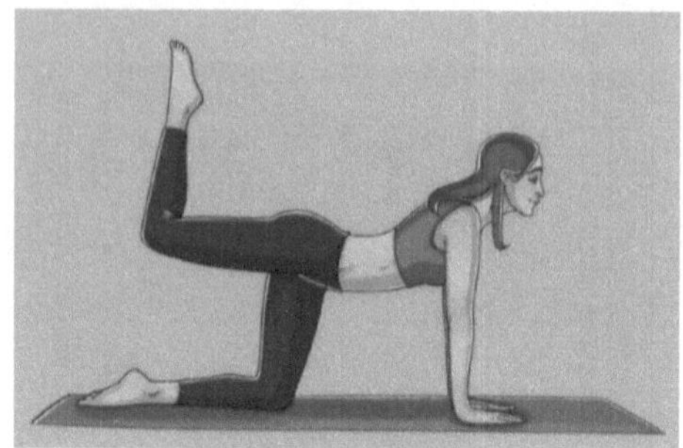

(brightside)

- Start with on all fours, your arms are below right under your shoulders.
- Keep one leg at 90 degree angle while lifting the other leg up to the air.
- You should not lift your thigh over your back much. How it works depending on your form, not your speed.
- When lowering it down, try to keep your knee off the floor and your leg is still 90 degree angle.

Side-lying leg lift (thighs, glutes)

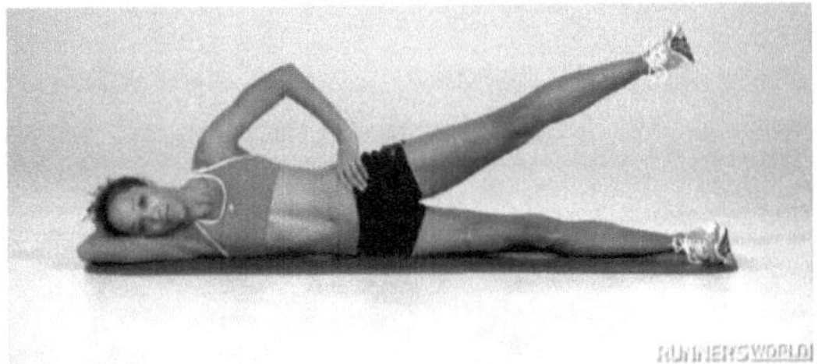

(youtube)

- Your body is in a straight line.

- Lift one leg and squeeze your belly for a while before lowering it down.

- While lowering it to the initial position, you should not touch the other leg until your workout time's done.

Superman (lower back, glute)

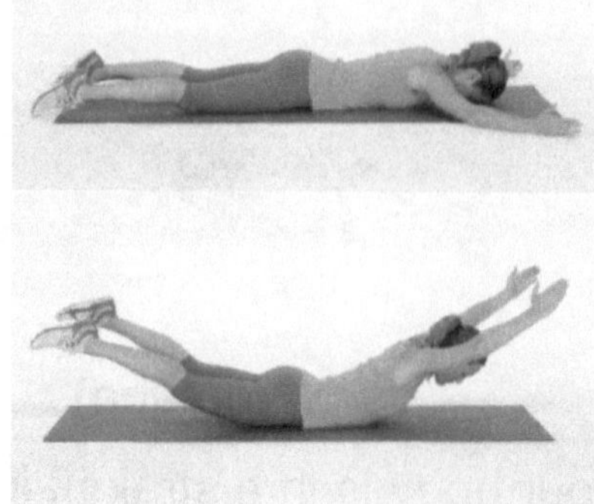

(posugar)

- Lift your legs and arms toward the ceiling. Keep this pose for a few seconds before lowering down.

- Inhale when you're facing down and exhale when you lift up.

Standing elbow to knee crunch (lower body)

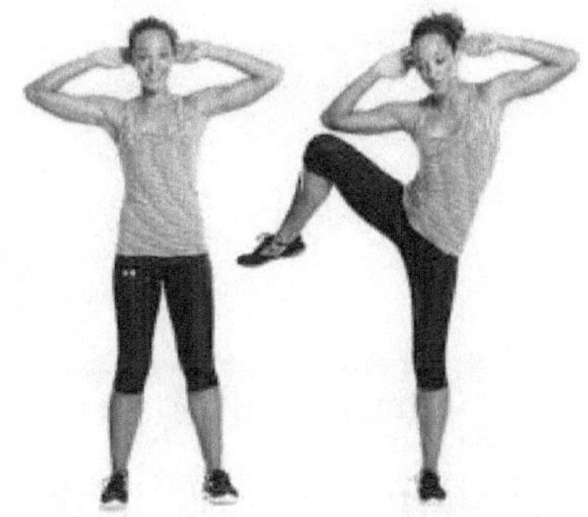

(pinterest)

- Squeeze your belly while lifting your knees so it can touch your elbows.
- Make sure you don't put pressure on your neck. Keep it at the neutral position.

Abs bicycle (oblique abs)

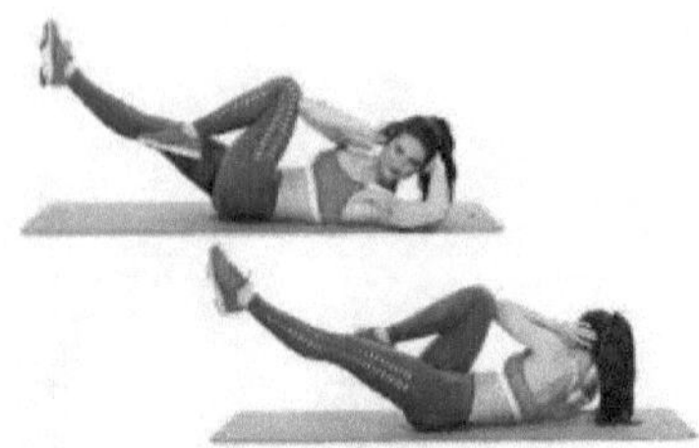

(trainwithkhaled.com)

- Bring your legs as high as you can (about 30-45 degrees). Touch your elbows with your knees alternatively.

- Your belly should feel a litle stressed or extended.

Plank jack (abs)

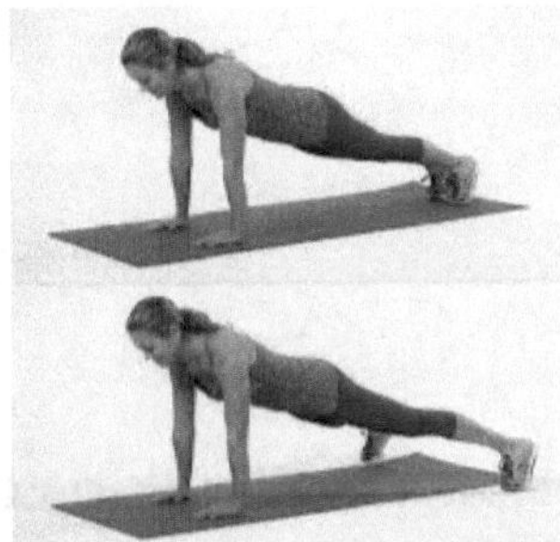

(popsugar)

- Your arms are straight under your shoulders. Start with the high plank position then try to jump on the spot by moving your legs.

- It is like you just move your lower body, your legs are kept slightly straight or you can loosen them a little bit so that you don't push yourself too much.

- Jump your feet out far your shoulders then put them back again to the initial position.

Flutter kick (abs, legs)

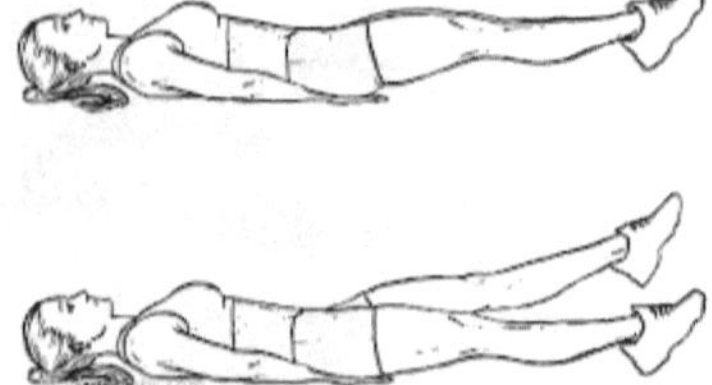

(workoutlabs.com)

- Move up and down while keeping your legs straight.
- You can move as low as you would like but make sure they are not touching the floor.

Scissor kick (abs, legs)

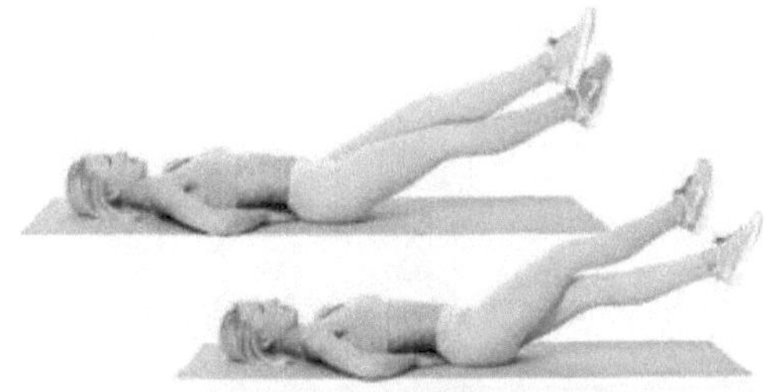

(trainhardteam.com)

- Move your legs left to right and alternatively.

- Put your hands behind your butt if you are quite unfamiliar with this exercise. Breathe normally.

Squat front kick (butt, abs)

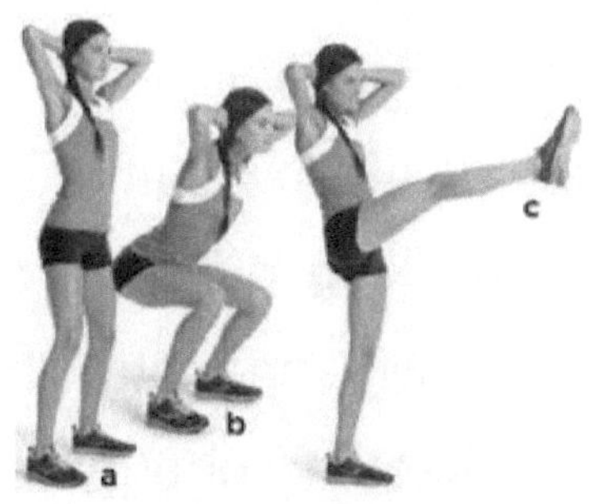

(pinterest)

After a squat pose, when you kick forward, keep your legs straight but not lock them.

Jump squat (legs, butt)

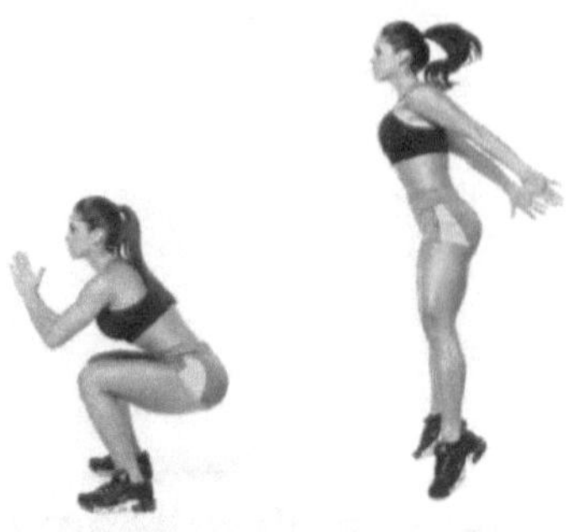

(oxygen magazine)

After doing a squat, jump off the floor while keeping your back straight.

You can choose workout targeting on certain muscle group or combining them like these sets:

For chest: cobra pose, dumbbell floor press.

For abs: plank, mountain climb.

For butt: squat, lie down-lift up.

After working out, you need to cool down your body slowly and stretch it a little bit for relaxing and keeping energy for the next working day.

During working out, you can have 20 seconds between every workout type to take a break for without being exhausted. Taking a deep

breath, drinking water slowly or lying down a little
bit for not push yourself too much pressure.

Chapter 6: Breathing techniques

Breathing techniques for losing belly fat

1. Morning breathing (belly breathing)

- Lie on back your mat or flat place. Bend your legs on the floor.

- Place your hands on your belly to control the right position.

- Slowly breathe in as much as you can while drawing your stomach strongly toward your spine so you can touch your ribs clearly (bring your stomach as close to your spine as possible).

- Hold this pose for 15-20 seconds.

- When you exhale, blow through your mouth energetically so you can feel all of the air go out your belly totally. You are aware of your breathing rhythm.

- Repeat 5 times.

Tips:

- When you do this technique remember to inhale through your nose and exhale through your mouth.

- You can do this anytime you'd like throughout the day. It works well when your stomach's empty (for example: in the morning, before going to bed). You can practice this deep breathing method while standing or sitting upright.

2. Qigong taught by Vietnamese physician Do Duc Ngoc[9]

- Lift your legs up to 45 degree. Hold them for 20 seconds while breathing normally without opening your mouth. Your head should be lifted up slightly (put your hands over it).

- Lift your legs down.

- Move your legs up and down gently while lifting up your head. Keep breathing without opening your mouth. This pose is also for 20 seconds.

- Move your legs from left to right and reverse while your head is lifted up, again while breathing normally and not opening your mouth. Do this pose for 20 seconds.

- Lie down, and breathe normally for 1 minute so that you feel slightly warm at your belly.

- Pull your left leg close to your chest, exhale strongly through mouth (like blowing a ballon) or like making a "whoosh" sound, then repeat with your right leg.

---

[9] Physician Do Duc Ngoc. https://khicongydaovietnam.wordpress.com/

- Keep doing this action for 50 seconds to 1 minute. Do this many times in a day, if you like.

3. Belly fat burning method using a towel taught by Japanese doctor Toshiki Fukutsudzi

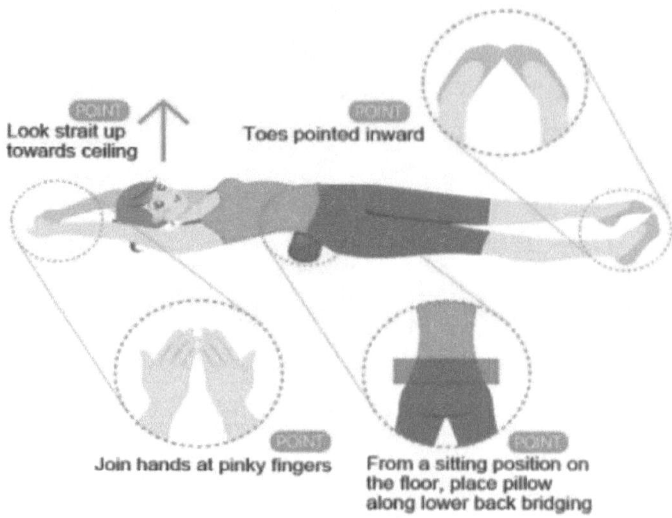

(healtified)

-   Tightly roll your towel so it is not less than 15 inches long (40 cm) and 4 inches wide (10cm).
-   Put it under your waist while lying down gently on your mat.
-   The towel must exactly be at under your navel. You can check it by moving your fingers from navel to towel under your waist.
-   Your legs are hip-width apart (about 3 inches or 8cm). Touch your big toes together. Keep your legs slightly straight.

100

- Stretch your arms over your head, palms down, try to touch your pinky fingers together.
- Breathe normally. Or you can breathe in for 3 seconds and breathe out for 7 seconds also. This works well too.
- Keep this pose for 5 minutes.
- Do this 3 times a day for the optimal result.
- When you finish this exercise, slowly sit up with no sudden jerking motion for not hurting your back.
- You should feel warm in your belly, if not, try to focus on your breathing progress. Keep track on your belly's 'flow of air'.
- It is hard at the beginning to keep this pose for 5 minutes, so you can start with a pace of 2-3 minutes, then increase gradually and do it as many times as you can.

4. Breathing while standing

-   For better digestion, you should stand up or walk around your room for 30 minutes after eating. This will take pressure off of your stomach and allow for better digestion of your meal.
-   Keep your chest up, flatten your belly while breathing normally.
-   You must not bend your back because it will make your belly fatter.

5. Lie down-lift up (good for abs, glutes, back pain killer)

- Lie on the mat with your face down

- Keep your hands close to your body and your legs straight and close together.

- Take a deep breath. Lift your upper body while holding breath as long as you can.

- Lie down again, exhale.

- Do this process 10-15 times a day, or many times as you like.

- Do this at least 3 days a week for the best result.

Stretching after workouts

Cobra stretch (shoulders, back, chest, abs, hips, and obliques)

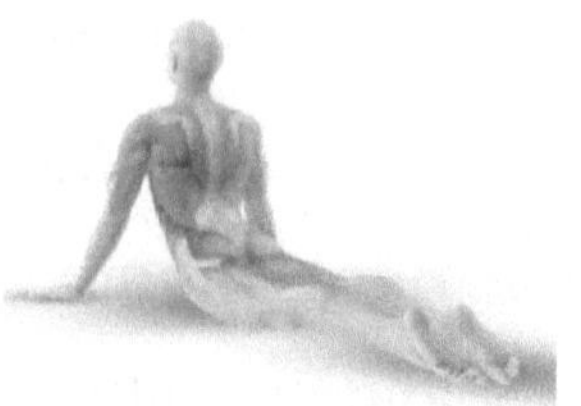

(brightside)

- Lie on your mat with your face down.
- Keep your hands close by your side and your feet close together.
- Lift your upper body up so you feel your belly is extended with your neck in a neutral position.
- Keep this pose for 20 seconds then repeat 2-3 times.

Child pose (lower back, hip, knee)

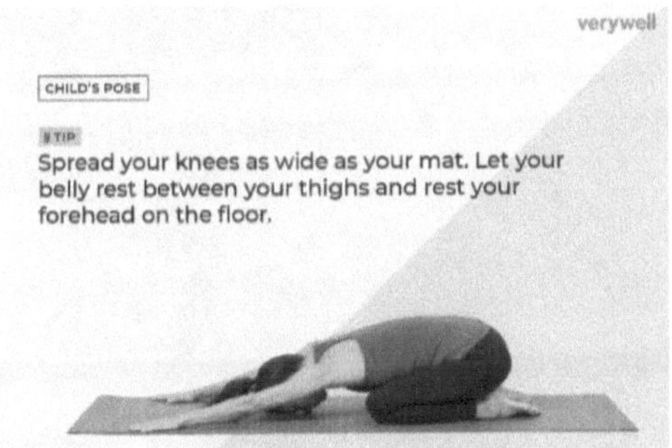

(verywell / ben goldstein)

- Kneel down keep your back straight, and put your hands on your thighs.
- Slightly slide your hands forward until your upper body touches the floor with your forehead down. Keep your chest touching your legs. Breathe deeply and slowly.
- Your arms are straight in front of you.
- Keep this pose for 20-30 seconds while breathing slowly. Do this 2 times.

Standing quadriceps stretch (legs)

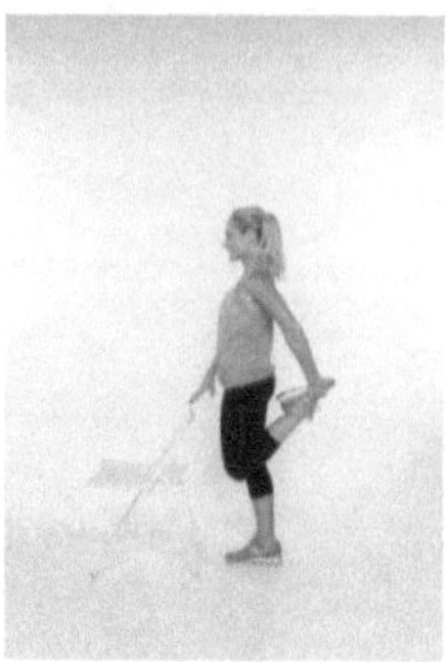

(myfitnesspalblog)

- Stand upright, you can hold a chair or touch the wall to keep your balance.
- Bent your left leg backward and hold your left ankle with your left hand.
- Keep this pose for 20 seconds.
- Similarly, do this for your right leg.
- Do this exercise 2-3 times or until you feel relaxed in your legs.

Lying trunk twist (belly)

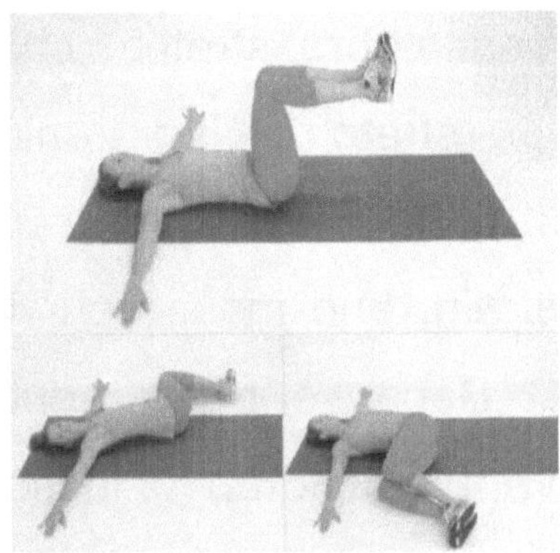

(popsugar)

- Lie on your mat, your shoulders should be on the floor.
- Raise your legs so they are at a 90 degrees angle with your upper body.
- Move them to the left side, your legs are close together.
- Keep this pose for 20-30 seconds.
- Then repeat for the right side.
- Do this exercise 2-3 times if possible.
- You might feel your oblique muscles extended

I tend to stretch my body after working out with 4 exercises: cobra stretch, child pose, standing quadriceps stretch, lying trunk twist more than twice as usual. It helps to prevent you from muscle strain, and make your workout day more beneficial. Because it can reduce muscle tension and prevent a build-up of lactic acid. Specialists believe that after workouts, stretching is essential and should never be skipped.

It is normal if you have pain in your muscles (or muscle soreness). It will appear within 24-48 hours after working out. For example, every time when I try another new exercise for my stubborn belly fat, I feel hurt in it within12-24 hours after working out. Wait until your body's dry, taking shower with warm water then cold water. It helps your muscles relax and you'll feel satisfied. Before and after taking a shower, drink a small cup of warm water or warm drink like tea for staying well hydrated. If you are unfamiliar with this pain, massage the damaging area by an analgesic ointment or just leave it. You will become this soreness after 2 weeks or more just by leaving it, ignoring it.

Making the habit of exercise is one part of your daily activity.

Consuming protein an hour after weight training helps your body repair damaged tissue and most effectively grow new tissue, said Thomas Goode, the doctor of naturopathy. A banana or a glass of milk is ideal also in this case.

Chapter 7. Losing weight by food

An extreme diet not only makes you feel nervous but also unintentionally gains weight. Make sure your intake is always less than output. If you want some light exercises like running, bicycle riding, and skipping, feel free to do them at anytime everyday. And also, remember to watch carefully to portion sizes. For example, when you were chubby, you ate 2 bowls of every kind of food or rice, now you should eat less day by day. Not keep it at bay but eat it with care.

As a demonstration, after 1 week, you can eat one and a half bowls of food. After 2 weeks, you can eat only 1 bowl. After 1 month, you can eat a little tiny bowl or a cup of food. When you get used to eating less for 1 month, you absolutely can eat less for your whole life.

Eat in moderation without starving yourself

Breakfast: homemade breakfasts are tasty and nutritious. You should eat an egg or drink a cup of milk. In my daily routine, I drink a cup of warm water first, then eat a bowl of porridge with pickled cucumber and 1 glass of soymilk.

Because high-protein food can help with weight management. One or two hours after breakfast, you should eat 1-2 jars of yogurt, they help your skin keep firm and smooth. Like Thomas Goode said you can break out of the lousy routine thus far described by consuming an adequate amount of protein in your breakfast meal. *Protein stimulates dopamine production, making you alert and active. You need protein in the morning to get you going and to keep you operating at your best. Also, consume protein as a major part of your meal before any afternoon or evening if you expect to be active.*

Do not skip breakfast as this will lead to a slow down in your metabolic rate and make it harder for you to lose weight. Skipping breakfast also puts pressure on the nervous system and will result in your body producing more adrenaline and cortisol – high levels of these two hormones make it harder biochemically for your body to metabolize fat and can lead to increased weight around the tummy area., wrote Rick Hay[10], the superfoodist.

---

[10] Rick Hay. The Anti Aging Food & Fitness Plan. 2016.

Midday: coffee, tea or warm water with honey

This is a great time of a day to maximize the fat burning qualities of caffeine.
Do not sweeten with sugar or artificial sweeteners – use half a teaspoon of honey if necessary. Or if you are busy, I recommend a cup of warm water with 1 teaspoon of honey. These drinks are good to help reduce bloating and fluid retention. They also stimulate liver function.

Another perspective on weight management is that the amount we are to eat is as individual was our bodies. Nature, in her wisdom, gives us a measure of how much we are to eat by the size of our hands.
Ideally we would only eat the amount we could hold in our cupped hands. One rounded handful is the quantity that is easily digestible for us.

Lunch: a tiny bowl of rice/ 1 cup of rice/ , meat/ fish (with moderation). 1 bowl of watery gruel.

Supper/ dinner: (try to eat before 6:30pm-7pm) you can choose fruit, cucumber, homemade food.

You should eat three meals a day. Three meals a day was the way of our modern ancestors. As for me, eating breakfast like a queen, lunch like a civilian and dinner like a super star model. Eating this way would mean that our digestive powers can grow with the sun when we eat the most – at breakfast. We should eat within an hour after rising. Each meal should be 3-4 hours apart, which gives your stomach time to digest food properly.

You can eat cucumbers, tomatoes anytime throughout the day. Be aware not to eat them together, you should eat them seperately to absorb their nutritions most. Eat them without counting quantities is not bad. Even a lousy meal filled with calories and fat will damage you.

Smart drinking

Stay away from soft drinks, sparkling water, energy drinks. If you really want these things and can't control yourself, you should drink them as slowly as possible. Hold it for a little while in your mouth, then swallow it with ease. Or you can pour 1/3 bottle of sparkling water into a glass of icy water, wait until all of the ice melts, and then you can drink it.

To make the diet routine become your daily habit you need some of your discipline, imagine about you future figure after successful diet. That thing will give you motivation to keep up.

Control your thoughts so you think like a person-have-healthy-weight if your goal is to reduce your size. What would he/she eat? How much would he/she have to eat? How would they exercise? Or even just stick to your goal, not compare yourself to another people because we are different since we were born.

Try drinking warm water throughout the day to help eliminate belly fat, reduce your appetite. You can still enjoy regular meals. Either mineral water or boiled water are good. Try not to drink cold or icy water. You can set alarm to remind your time of drinking water. Each 20 minutes will be good to drink a sip of water. And then you have enough water for a day.

The way you drink is important, too. This drink is a all day additional meal, so don't just throw it down.

Drink it slowly as if you were actually chewing and swallowing a meal.

If you're constipated, it's harder to lose weight – the banana provides fibre and energy that will boost you both physically and mentally.

Eat 1 or 2 bananas per day is a good way to release you from constipation.

Many of us consume less than the 48 to 64 ounces of water recommended each day. To lose weight by flushing fat from your system, increase your water intake so you are drinking 64 to 120 ounces per day. Compare it to priming a pump and getting water to flow through.

If you haven't ben getting enough water, your body has been retaining it. Drinking more water is actually the cure for water retention problems. The body has been holding on it because it needed it, wrote Thomas Goode, a naturopathic doctor .

Don't set your goal ambitiously.

Everyone starts from scratch, so does the weight loss progress. You can long for a fit body like celebrities who appear on the stages or magazines, but you also want to have a suitable weight altogether with your healthy mental and physical aspects. That's the genuine journey we all aim to reach. Just start by setting a goal everyday, like a mini game. For instance, if you can exercise everyday, 10 days in a row, it will be a success. If you can bike 5km to somewhere you like, it's a success too. Keep working patiently on your long-term goals day by day and stick to your journey.

Sleep quality

Sleeping is important for your diet routine. And you should get a goodnight's sleep everyday. Getting 7-9 hours of sleep a night is good for your body and brain. The national sleep foundation [11]re commended that we need to sleep between 7-9 hours at night. This is based on epidemiological evidence indicating that individuals who sleep under 6 hours or over 9 hours per night have a higher mortality rates than those who sleep 7-8 hours per night. The lack of sleep has also been associated with higher BMI. That means if you sleep well, you can achieve your weight loss goal easier than who don't. Not sleeping well makes you gain weight at uncontrollable speed also.

Go to bed at least 3 hours after dinner and don't keep your phone close to you. I had a nightmare when I let it behind my ear, under my

---

[11] Cynthia A. Thomson, Kelly L. Morrow, Shirley W. Flatt, Betsy C. Wertheim, Michelle M. Perfect, Jennifer J. Ravia, Nancy E. Sherwood, Njeri Karanja, and Cheryl L. Rock. Relationship Between Sleep Quality and Quantity and Weight Loss in Women Participating in a Weight-Loss Intervention Trial.
https://www.ncbi.nlm.nih.gov/pmc/articles/PMC4861065/

pillow. And it made me dream all night about something I was scared of. The day after was a disaster. So, you had all day to use your smartphone, just let it go by putting it away from you or turning off at night for your optimal health and for its resting duration.

You should go to bed before 10pm and sleep heavily from 12 am to 2am. Sleep tight in darkness. 20 minutes before you go to sleep, you should turn off your lamp and all of electrical devices.

According to Thomas Goode, ND, *sleep is important in weight management because we need time to recover from the stress of living. Here are some tips to help you get the the sleep possible:*

- *Arise at the same time each day – even if you got less sleep than you wanted. A regular schedule is the best sleep aid.*
- *Keep your bedroom dark, quiet and cool. Watching TV in the bedroom is a sleep killer.*
- *Go to bed when you are sleepy. If you don't fall asleep within thirty minutes, get out of bed.*
- *Limit naps to under ½ hour maximum. Eliminate them if they keep you from sleeping.*
- *Exercise regularly and avoid caffeine for at least 5 hours before bedtime.*

I usually drink a cup of warm water before going to bed to stay hydrated and to get a good night sleep.

Practive belly breathing before going to bed is a good idea to sleep better. Breathe in through your nose without thinking about anything, and let your mind blank. Breathe in deeply so you feel your belly is swelling. Breathe out by your belly and you feel your belly flattens. Repeat this slowly until you fall asleep. Doing child pose is also an alternative way to sleep better.

Time to say goodbye to my first readers

The ten steps for weight loss and anti-aging

1. Identify your ideal weight

2. Set a goal to reach it with many small steps.

3. Visualize reaching your goal as you practice deep breathing or belly breathing, feel it and make it real in your mind-body.

4. Drink diluted lemon juice and turmeric warm water daily.

5. Smile everyday, let yourself soak in positive thoughts.

6. Avoid unnatural foods.

7. Eat in moderation.

8. Exercise regularly, sweat joyfully.

9. Double cleansing at the end of a day.

10. Use retinol at night.

Losing weight and keeping your face young may seem like an impossible dream, but it is possible if you really work hard at it. Adding a pinch of good humor also helps a lot. Andrey Hepburn once said "nothing is impossible" and that "the word itself says, I'm possible". This is fitting quote when it comes to losing weight. It doesn't matter if you srat point is 60, 100 or 200 kg or more, if you believe in it you can make it happen.

Losing weight is not the final goal but the beginning of happy journey instead.

If you are told you're ugly, fat and stupid, try your best to be more beautiful, get fit and be more knowledgable than the person who insulted you. If you lose weight successfully, it would be the sweetest fruit for yourselves trying. And also it might be a knock out to whom insulted you. If you can do it, you will be a better person for a better day of yourselves.

For my part, losing weight saved my life. It helped boost my confidence and stop body shame myself. It proved to me that I can do anything that seems impossible using only my strong willpower. It gave me strength in mental and physical health. You and I, we were born to shine!

Would you do me a favor?

If you like this book or have some suggestions for me, please leave reviews on Amazon. Inquiries are welcome. Questions may be sent directly to chithailan66@gmail.com. I'll appreciate all of your opinions. Thank you.

Reference resource

1. Rick Hay. The Anti Aging Food & Fitness Plan. 2016.

2. Thomas Goode,ND. The holistic guide to weightloss, anti-aging and fat prevention. 2005.

3. Allison Tannis, MS., R.H.N. FEED YOUR SKIN, STARVE YOUR WRINKLES. : Eat Your Way to Firmer, More Beautiful Skin with 100 Foods That Turn Back the Clock. 2009

4. Tiffany Mccoy. 100lbs.later. "How I lost over 100lbs.in 8 months and How YOU Can Do It Too!. 2015.

Https://www.popsugar.com/fitness/How-Do-Superman-Exercise-1110085

https://brightside.me/inspiration-health/a-5-week-workout-that-can-transform-your-body-like-a-magic-spell-730310/

https://www.bollywoodshaadis.com/articles/japanese-weight-loss-technique-6932

https://www.quora.com/Does-the-Japanese-technique-of-weight-loss-using-a-towel-work

https://redhousespice.com/egg-drop-soup/

https://timesofindia.indiatimes.com/life-style/food-news/turmeric-and-honey-two-powerful-antibiotics-even-doctors-cant-explain/photostory/68111462.cms?Picid=68111466

https://www.sciencedirect.com/topics/medicine-and-dentistry/curcuminoid

https://www.ncbi.nlm.nih.gov/pmc/articles/PMC5424551/

https://www.healthline.com/nutrition/top-10-evidence-based-health-benefits-of-turmeric#section8

https://www.rasmussen.edu/degrees/health-sciences/blog/surprising-health-benefits-of-donating-blood/

https://brightside.me/inspiration-health/12-stretches-you-can-do-at-home-to-burn-fat-471060/

https://www.huffpost.com/entry/not-overeating_b_969910

https://www.popsugar.com/fitness/photo-gallery/33387812/image/33716237/Trunk-Twist

https://www.drworkout.fitness/leg-press-foot-placement-variations/

https://classpass.com/movements/tricep-extension

https://www.medicalnewstoday.com/articles/324585#lemon-juice

https://www.bulletproof.com/supplements/aminos-enzymes/digestive-enzymes-guide/

https://www.womenshealthmag.com/uk/fitness/workouts/a702091/how-to-do-a-dumbbell-floor-press/